P9-APP-046

i

A Pound of Cure

Change Your Eating and Your Life, One Step at a Time

by

Matthew Weiner, MD, FACS

To Loren, Lucy, & Ruby – My first station.

Copyright © 2013 by Matthew Weiner, MD
All rights reserved. No part of this book may be reproduced,
scanned, or distributed in any printed or electronic form without
permission.

First Edition: January 2013
Printed in the United States of America
ISBN: 978-1-14810611-4-8

This book is not intended to replace advice from a physician. If you have any medical conditions or symptoms that are concerning, a physician should be consulted, rather than relying on the information found within this book. This book represents the current state of medical knowledge as of November 2012. As more research becomes available, some of the information in this book may become invalid. You should seek the most up to date information from a physician or other health care professional.

Table of Contents

ACKNOWLEDGEMENTS

This book would not have been possible without the love and support of my beautiful wife, Loren. Besides the patience and flexibility that any surgeon's wife must possess, Loren has been instrumental in implementing the *Pound of Cure* plan in our household. The recipes are her work (except for a few from my mother) and represent her creative, yet pragmatic approach to cooking.

My office manager, Carol Finkelstein also deserves credit for her role as a sounding board for many of the ideas contained in this book. Her hard work, intelligence, and efficiency have been critical to our success thus far.

I'd also like to acknowledge the work of Joel Fuhrman, MD, and Lee Kaplan, MD, PhD whose ideas and research keyed me into the power of fruits and vegetables and the role of the body's set point in weight loss, respectively.

Finally, I'd like to thank my patients who have trusted me over the years and had faith in my abilities. The cumulative sum of your stories has inspired me to develop the *Pound of Cure* eating plan.

Introduction

Although the United States is one of the most powerful nations in the world, there is one area where we lag way behind the rest of the world – nutrition. Our food chain is incredibly efficient at delivering calories to Americans. We've nearly eliminated starvation in our country and even the poorest individuals still receive more than enough calories to survive. However, the United States is entirely *deficient* at delivering nutrients to Americans. A trip to any grocery store in the country can demonstrate this fact clearly. The produce section, which contains the foods with the most nutrients, typically takes up only a small portion of the store. However, the breakfast cereals, desserts, potato chips, soda pop, and bread products take up the vast majority of the shelf space.

Obesity is not a disease of gluttony as most people think – it is a disease of metabolism. All of us know someone of normal weight who eats large amounts of junk food daily yet manages to stay thin. The vast majority of Americans subsist largely on processed foods, yet only a third of us develop significant obesity. The reason that only some people gain significant amounts of weight has to do with how our body reacts to these foods. Those who suffer from obesity are triggered to store processed foods as fat while those who remain free of obesity are not nearly as efficient at fat storage. If you are significantly overweight, chances are you are more susceptible to processed foods than others. It is not the calories contained in processed food that make them so fattening. It is the intrinsic, less measurable properties of these foods that alter your metabolism more than they do your skinnier friends. Long term weight loss depends on limiting processed foods and replacing them with large amounts of nutritious food for the rest of your life - and no less. The *Pound of Cure* eating plan will help you to accomplish this difficult task.

The relationship between processed foods and obesity is very similar to the development of lung cancer or emphysema after years of smoking cigarettes. Some smokers develop lung cancer and die in their fifties and sixties, while others live well into their eighties, never severely affected by their tobacco habits. The solution to lung cancer is not to figure out how to make all smokers react to tobacco like those who live into their eighties. The solution is to eliminate smoking. The same is true for obesity. To address America's weight problem, we need to minimize processed foods in our diet and replace them with foods that are rich in nutrients.

Your Metabolic Thermostat

Weight loss is a very difficult undertaking as anyone more than a few pounds overweight can attest to. The reason that weight loss is so difficult and weight gain comes on so easily is due to a metabolic principle that I refer to as the "thermostat effect." Just as a thermostat works to balance the amount of cold and warm air that is pushed into a room to maintain a constant temperature, our metabolism has a built in "thermostat" that works to adjust the balance between the calories that are burned and consumed to keep your body weight constant. This metabolic thermostat works to keep our weight from dropping too low regardless of the environmental conditions. Believe it or not, the thermostat also works to keep us from overeating and gaining too much weight. Durable weight loss does not come from eating fewer calories; it comes from re-setting your thermostat to a lower weight and maintaining this setting.

This theory stands directly against the widely accepted model of obesity that claims that weight gain is the result of eating too much and exercising too little. The medical community and popular press have embraced the idea that obesity is the result of gluttonous eating and sloth like behavior. This belief has spawned an extensive network of diet programs designed to alter behavior through meticulous point or calorie counting, exercise programs, convenient portion controlled meals, and even hypnotism targeted at blocking hunger. These programs uniformly fail - not due to the lack of discipline of the participants, but because the fundamental philosophy behind them is deeply flawed.

It is only after performing hundreds of gastric bypass procedures that I recognized the holes in the behavioral model of obesity. I have watched closely as surgical patients lost weight easily and permanently while others tried and failed through one form of starvation or another. The research that debates the validity of these two competing models of weight loss is extensive and complex. So, please be patient with me over these next few pages as I try to explain why a short circuit in our metabolic thermostat is a more accurate model for obesity.

Let's start with a simple fact – one pound of fat contains approximately 3,500 calories. It doesn't matter if the fat comes from lard or vegetable oil, it contains 3,500 calories. This also means that in order to lose one pound of body fat, you must burn 3,500 more calories than you take in.

Now, let's look at how many extra calories a 50-year-old man who weighs 400 pounds must eat, assuming he was

150 pounds at age 15. Using the standard model of calories in versus calories out, you'll find that it takes less than 70 extra calories per day to cause someone to gain 250 pounds over the first half of their adult life. One slice of bread contains 70 calories, so the 400 pound, 50-year-old man, that is judged by society to be a glutton and a sloth, has committed the egregious sin of eating one extra slice of bread every day. This also assumes that if you have been able to maintain your weight over your adult life, you have done it by consciously altering your food intake to match your energy expenditure down to the last crumb, because even 10 extra calories a day will result in an extra pound added every year.

The fact that anyone can manage to stay thin proves that maintaining an equal calorie balance is not a cognitive exercise but rather a subconscious one, just like maintaining a constant respiratory or heart rate. Since we must acknowledge that there are subconscious controls that impact the tight balance between calories consumed and calories expended, we can only assume that obesity is the result of an alteration of the control system.

Under starvation conditions (or during a diet), we typically lose a few pounds rapidly causing our current weight to drop several pounds below our metabolic thermostat's set point. After a few weeks of starvation, our metabolic thermostat kicks in to try to remedy this abnormality. Many people assume that losing weight triggers our metabolism to slow down – this is correct, but only partially so. To get a complete understanding of why traditional starvation diets fail, we must look at the different ways our metabolic thermostat controls our calorie balance.

The first and most effective way that our body will remedy the discrepancy between our starved weight and our metabolic thermostat's set point is to release hormones that trigger our brain to seek out food. Many people think that resisting food temptations while on a diet is a matter of willpower and that their inability to resist the temptations of food is a sign of mental weakness. The situation is so much more complex than that! You are much less in charge of your ability to resist food temptations than you think. After a few weeks on a traditional starvation diet, your brain is flooded with hormones that drive you to eat more.

Your brain will also release neurotransmitters that cause you to move slower and expend less energy. You will find yourself sitting down more often and dodging phone calls from your workout partner. In short, starvation will cause your brain to transform you from the willing, determined person that started your diet into a glutton and a sloth – and there is not much that you can do about it. Please don't misinterpret this last statement – it does not mean that there is nothing that you can do about your weight. It only means that you cannot starve the weight off through traditional diets.

The best example of the behavioral changes that food deprivation can cause comes from the Minnesota Starvation Experiment carried out between 1944 and 1945. In this experiment, healthy volunteers were forced to eat a very low calorie diet for almost an entire year and the physical and psychological effects were measured.

The study was carried out primarily on conscientious objectors of the war who volunteered for the study as an alternative to military service. The subjects were thoroughly screened for any pre-existing medical or psychiatric conditions.

During the study period, depression, anxiety, and severe emotional distress were observed. Also, the subjects exhibited an obsession with food and developed long, drawn out eating rituals for their meager portions. Often, the subjects were observed swapping recipes with each other and recalling their favorite meals or other events centered on food.

The subjects also became extremely lazy. They started sleeping excessively and their personalities became more introverted. The subjects reported that they all knew where the elevators were and would avoid the stairwells as much as possible.

Many people assume that their ability to endure prolonged, restrictive diets is merely a matter of willpower. But, the Minnesota Starvation Experiment reveals that our desire to eat is primal and powerful and will eventually overcome even the most disciplined minds. Just as willpower cannot be used to hold your breath to the point of suffocation, following a calorie-restricted diet forever is impossible once your hunger drive takes over.

So if traditional starvation diets will never work, what can be done to lose the weight and keep it off? The answer is to learn how to re-set our metabolic thermostat to a lower weight. The *Pound of Cure* diet was created for this purpose exactly.

Everyone's thermostat is set to a different weight by a combination of both environmental and genetic factors. This explains why your sister-in-law who eats a dozen donuts weekly stays thin while you manage to gain a few pounds just from walking into a bakery. As you age, there are many events that can increase the setting on your thermostat. Pregnancy, processed foods, menopause, certain medications and an injury that results in a prolonged period of decreased physical activity can all set your thermostat to a new, higher weight. If your metabolic thermostat is turned up, you will become just like the subjects in the Minnesota Starvation Experiment. You will develop insatiable hunger and will avoid physical activity at all costs. You will be powerless to resist the additional pounds that you pack on as your metabolic thermostat drives your current weight up to its new, higher setting.

We've examined the changes in your brain and your body that occur when you starve yourself below your thermostat's setting. Now let's look at the opposite situation - when you are overfed up to a weight that exceeds your thermostat's setting. Very few studies examine the effects of overfeeding on humans, however, there are dozens of studies in rats.

When rats are overfed by using a feeding tube to deliver twice as many calories as rats typically consume, they gain weight. It is not surprising that they gain more weight than rats who are allowed to eat freely. This experiment alone is hardly ground breaking. The interesting results come after the feeding tube is removed and the rats are allowed to eat freely again. The overfed rats will move more frequently and naturally eat less than the rats who were allowed to eat normally during the entirety of the experiment. After a few weeks, the weights of the overfed rats will slowly drift downward to match the weights of the other group of rats. When a rat is overfed, its current weight is artificially driven above its metabolic thermostat's set point. When this happens, the results are equal and opposite to those that occur after a period of starvation. The rats lose their appetite and begin to eat less. They also move more in an effort to burn additional calories and shift their body weight back toward the lower set point.

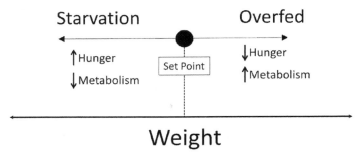

Figure 1 - Your metabolic thermostat

We see very similar changes in humans who stop taking medications that increase their metabolic thermostat's setting. The best example is the temporary use of corticosteroids like Prednisone. Corticosteroids work to decrease inflammation and are used to treat conditions like Crohn's disease and Rheumatoid Arthritis. When a patient is placed on these medications, they gain weight because corticosteroids work to increase your metabolic thermostat's set point. Once the medications are stopped, the thermostat goes back down to its original setting, leaving the patient in an "overfed" state. The patient will lose their appetite, begin moving more frequently, and the weight will naturally drift back down to the original set point.

Long term weight loss success lies in learning how to reset your thermostat to a lower weight. The *Pound of Cure* diet is different from traditional restrictive diets that limit your calorie intake and rely on self-imposed periods of starvation that will never result in durable weight loss. It is only by changing the content of your diet that you can hope to nudge your thermostat down to a healthier weight. This can only be done slowly, over time, utilizing a diet that is rich in nutrients, unlimited in portions, and makes no attempts to thwart your hunger drive. Over the period of a year or even more, the excess fat will disappear as your thermostat is reset to a healthier weight.

Resetting Your Thermostat

The best known way to lower your body's metabolic thermostat is to undergo bariatric (weight loss) surgery. Much of the research that supports the thermostat set point model of weight loss comes from observing the biochemical changes that occur after bariatric surgery. As a bariatric surgeon, who also provides weight loss counseling in my practice, I noticed a profound difference between patients who were losing weight as the result of a surgical procedure and those suffering through starvation diets. The gastric bypass procedure works to immediately change your thermostat set point to a much lower level. All of the typical metabolic and hormonal changes that occur while on a starvation diet occur in exactly the opposite direction after bariatric surgery.

As we've discussed, starvation diets cause your metabolism and body movements to slow down. After bariatric surgery, metabolism and body movements increase despite the fact that the patient is eating very few calories and should be exhibiting metabolic signs of starvation. I refer to the increased body movements seen after surgery as the "gastric bypass swagger." The still obese post-surgical patient begins to walk a little differently with exaggerated arm and shoulder movements, and longer strides.

Starvation diets trigger the release of hormones that stimulate hunger, causing us to become obsessed with food, just as we saw in the Minnesota Starvation Experiment. For six months or more after surgery, bariatric patients report little to no hunger and several experiments have documented much lower blood levels of several hunger inducing hormones.

The reasons for the lack of hunger and increased metabolism seen after surgery now becomes clear when viewed through a "set point" lens. A gastric bypass procedure immediately resets your body's metabolic thermostat to a much lower level. The result is that the post-surgical patient is immediately converted into an overfed state and will decrease their desire for food and increase their body movements to reduce their weight down to this new, lower setting. It is for these reasons that bariatric surgery offers success rates that are 10-20 times higher than those seen after a program of restrictive dieting and exercise.

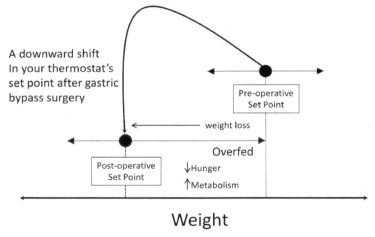

Figure 2 - Weight loss after gastric bypass surgery

The understanding that bariatric surgery induces weight loss primarily through the immediate and substantial lowering of your metabolic thermostat begs the obvious question – are there any other ways that we can lower our thermostat's set point? It turns out that indeed, there are and this provides an opportunity to offer a much-improved alternative to traditional starvation diets.

It comes as no surprise that your thermostat's setting can be altered by medications. Some medications, like the corticosteroids we previously discussed will increase your thermostat's set point and cause you to gain weight rapidly. Insulin injections, used to treat diabetes, can have the same effect and the role of insulin in modulating your metabolic thermostat will be discussed later. Other medications, like Phentermine (a diet pill that made up the second half of Fen-Phen when it was on the market) can shift it a few pounds downward and is an effective weight loss drug. Patients report, that while taking Phentermine, they naturally ate less and lost weight very easily. They also report feeling very "jittery" and having difficulty sleeping while on the medication - further demonstrating that when your current weight exceeds your metabolic thermostat's setting, your body will increase your physical movement in order to burn off the "excess" calories. Unfortunately, Phentermine has a troubling side effect profile and you cannot stay on it for long periods of time. Additionally, as soon as you stop taking the drug, your thermostat will go right back to its original setting, resulting in weight regain. Nicotine is another drug that can lower your thermostat which explains why many people gain weight rapidly after they quit smoking. Clearly the side effects of tobacco and nicotine prohibit its use as safe weight loss agent. At this time, there are no medications that can safely reduce your thermostat's set point and I do not use drug therapy in my practice.

A far better way to lower your thermostat is to increase the amount of healthy muscle that you have. This is a very difficult task for many people due to physical limitations, age, and available time. As we age we lose muscle. This process starts at a frustratingly young age. The result of the early onset of muscle loss is that there is not much that most of us can do to build up a substantial amount of muscle. This explains the relatively small impact of exercise on lowering our thermostat.

The final - and most important - way that you can lower your thermostat is to change the types of food that you eat. When we look more closely at our metabolic thermostat, we find that there are built in sensors in our body that determine whether we are on the starved or overfed side of our set point. As bariatric surgery demonstrates, the most important sensors are located in our gastrointestinal (GI) tract; primarily in our stomach and small intestines. A gastric bypass procedure rearranges the flow of nutrients through the GI tract, altering the signals that these sensors send back to the brain's thermostat. We can cause a similar change to the signals being sent back to our brain by our stomach and small intestines by altering the types of food that we eat. It's important that it is the types of food, not the amount that is important. The effects of food take much longer to work than those caused by a surgical rearrangement, but can ultimately be just as powerful.

First and foremost, the *Pound of Cure* eating plan was designed to encourage the intake of large amounts of food that lower your thermostat's set point. It will also point out those foods that we've been convinced make good diet choices, but actually work to raise our thermostat's set point. Because of the slow and gradual effect of food on your thermostat, your long term success can only be determined over seasons or even longer. If you manage to eat large amounts of natural, thermostat lowering foods, and limit your consumption of processed, thermostat raising foods to only a few times a week, you will nudge your set point down a little bit every day. Only by lowering your thermostat's set point can you hope to lose weight without experiencing binge-inducing hunger and weight loss plateaus from a slowed metabolism.

Changing Tastes

The *Pound of Cure* program will teach you how to gradually improve the quality of your diet, shifting away from processed foods toward thermostat lowering fruits and vegetables. Because the average American's diet consists primarily of processed foods, our taste buds have adapted to the sweet, salty, rich tastes of today's foods. After years of eating like this, healthy, natural foods are unable to stimulate our taste buds in a meaningful way causing them to be interpreted as "tasteless." Even the sweetest strawberries will taste bland to people who regularly drink sweetened strawberry milkshakes or eat strawberry ice cream. Over time, we've developed tolerance to sweet, salty, and rich tastes that require even stronger tastes to satisfy us.

Thankfully, these changes are not permanent and can be reversed over a period of about six months. As you wean yourself from the American diet, you'll begin to derive the same pleasure from fruits and vegetables that you do from your current diet. Many people doubt this statement, but I've seen it happen hundreds of times. Eventually, the taste of a strawberry shake will be interpreted as "too sweet," unless you return to drinking them regularly. The delicious tastes of natural foods are masked by commercial sweetening, salting, and frying processes. Once you eliminate the processed foods from your diet, you'll begin to enjoy the natural tastes of fruits, vegetables, nuts, seeds, eggs, poultry, fish, and meats.

Controlling Hunger

The commercial foods prevalent in our modern diet stimulate our cravings for more sweet, salty, and rich tastes. In fact, they're designed for just this purpose. As you move toward a more natural diet, you'll find that the intense cravings you have at meal times and in the evening will diminish. Furthermore, eating large amounts of fruits and vegetables will provide ample amounts of micronutrients. Although micronutrients typically refer to the vitamins and minerals that are necessary for health, they also include the thousands of undiscovered compounds that are so vital to our health and help to prevent chronic diseases. If your body is no longer starved of these micronutrients, you will experience less hunger throughout the day.

Most patients on this program report that their food cravings are decreased after just a few days and almost completely eliminated after 2-4 weeks. This is approximately the time that it takes to detox from processed foods. Ultimately, after 6 months of eating using the *Pound of Cure* method, you'll find that if you do fall back to your old eating style, you will develop nausea and fatigue. It's at this point that you realize you used to feel like this all day long!

The *Pound of Cure* eating method is perfect for those people who love to cook and love to eat. In fact, this is exactly the type of person who succeeds on this program. The cooking skills that you have developed over the years are integral to your success on this program. The only thing that will change is the ingredient list. Ultimately, you'll begin to enjoy the tastes of natural foods as much as you enjoy the sweet, salty, creamy tastes that you favor today.

This program is designed to help you change the way you eat in a slow, methodical fashion in an attempt to make you a healthier person and lower your metabolic thermostat. Exercise makes up only a very small portion of the program and is not necessary for your success. Also, this program is as much about what you DO eat as what you DON'T. We start by adding in foods that lower your thermostat's set point and eventually eliminate the ones that cause weight gain by raising your set point. After you add in the healthy foods, it will be much easier to remove the unhealthy ones.

The Commercial Diet Industry

The *Pound of Cure* is an entirely non-commercial weight loss program - it is not driven or developed to reap profits or sell products. It provides only information about the healthiest foods and instructions on how to incorporate them into your diet. The diet industry is approaching $100 billion dollars per year and nearly every commercial program is profit driven, rather than health driven. Most programs rely heavily on their own proprietary foods, snacks, shakes, powders, and pills as part of the magic that results in weight loss. These programs typically require only small changes and result in modest, temporary weight loss – just enough to convince you that it is your fault, not the program's that you ultimately fail and regain the weight. They will not change your body's thermostat set point and will merely induce a period of starvation that will slow your metabolism and increase your hunger. In order to succeed and reach your goal of life long weight loss and health, you must reject the low fat, low calorie, and low carbohydrate mantras of the commercial diet industry. The small tweaks in your diet to lower calorie versions of processed food that the commercial diet industry pedals are not enough to cause durable weight loss. Permanent, significant weight loss requires major and substantial changes to your eating. The *Pound of Cure* eating method will show you how to gradually make these changes in your life.

Success is not achieved by replacing high-calorie refined foods with even more refined low-fat, low-carbohydrate, and low-calorie versions. These "diet" foods are nearly as dangerous as their full-fat and full-sugar counterparts are and are not a part of your successful weight loss formula. Rather, our goal is to eliminate your desire for all processed foods by eating large amounts of fruits and vegetables that are "nutrient dense" – high in nutrition but low in calories.

How to Measure Success

You will lose weight – perhaps lots of it, but the scale cannot be our primary determinant of success. Instead, we will focus our energy on your habits, attitudes, and behaviors about food, knowing that in the long run, this will result in weight loss. Using the scale as a measurement of success or failure is forbidden. If your primary goal is to lose weight, I recommend you weigh yourself no more frequently than once a month - ideally only once a season. Rather than determining your success by the number on the scale, measure your success by your eating habits. If you are eating well, following the program, trying out new recipes and slowly changing your attitudes about food, consider yourself a success.

Some weeks you may lose weight. Others, you may not. This does not mean that you were more successful during the weeks that you lost weight. Your body's metabolism is a very unpredictable machine if you look at it day by day. You may lose weight at times you are not eating your best and may not lose weight during the times when you're most compliant. Weight loss should be looked at over months, or even seasons. Only over longer time periods will your eating changes be accurately reflected by the scale.

In my practice, I see patients with anywhere from 5-500 pounds to lose. I perform weight loss surgery and also use non-surgical techniques to assist patients in weight loss. The *Pound of Cure* eating program was designed to offer patients who either do not qualify for or do not wish to undergo bariatric surgery a method for driving down your body's thermostat to allow for permanent, lifelong weight loss.

Regardless of your current eating habits, the slow, methodical modification in your diet that you are about to make will improve your health, help you conquer your cravings for processed foods, and decrease your waistline dramatically. This program contains twelve "stations" or changes that you can progress through as quickly or as slowly as you like. It's probably better to dwell for a month (if not longer) on each station to make sure you fully integrate each change into your life. If you move too fast you may not fully embrace each change and fail to maximize its potential. Also, food will not cause a rapid change in your thermostat set point the way bariatric surgery does. Because of this, there is little benefit in making drastic changes quickly; you can lose weight just as effectively if you gradually implement each station over time, slowly nudging your thermostat downward.

As you progress through each station you will start to look at the way you used to eat (and others continue to eat) in an enlightened fashion - finally recognizing the damage to your health that most of today's processed foods cause.

Portion Control is Not Necessary

The *Pound of Cure* eating plan makes no stipulations about portion control for most foods. In fact, it is specifically designed to not cause calorie restriction which triggers your thermostat to slow your metabolism down and increase your hunger drive. You should eat heartily when you are hungry until you are satisfied. Most of the foods that you are eating will promote weight loss rather than weight gain so you can eat as much as you want, at any time of day. As your health improves and eating habits become more engrained,

17

you will find that eating thermostat lowering foods naturally decreases your portion size.

There is a rationale for the order of the stations – each step teaches you techniques that better enable you to reach the next station. This order works well for most, but not all patients. You should not feel obligated to move through them in the exact order they are presented. **Minor** modifications are acceptable.

There is no need to progress through all twelve stations. In fact, most patients don't. Since the impact of this program varies from person to person, you may find that your health goals can be met by applying just the first five stations. You may also find that it is only necessary to partially integrate certain stations. This is also acceptable. If the only change you make is to incorporate Station 2 (1 pound of vegetables daily) into your everyday life, this alone will result in significant health benefits and perhaps a little bit of weight loss over time. The choice is yours as to how far you want to take this.

Good Nutrition is For Life

It's critical to realize that this program is never intended to end. As you move through each station, you should consider it a permanent change. Once you start eating one pound of vegetables daily, the understanding is that you will continue this behavior forever. Until the behavior changes stipulated in a station are part of your daily routine, you should not move on to the next station. This is intended to be a journey that continues for the remainder of your life, rather than a program with a beginning and an end. In short, this book aims to provide you the tools necessary for a lifetime of good health.

The Metabolic Reset Program

Daily Food Plan:

Protein: Limit to 3 servings for women, 4 servings for men
  1 serving MUST be a vegetable protein
Vegetables: AT LEAST 1 pound daily, but enjoy unlimited servings
Fruit: Unlimited (avoid canned fruits)
Fats: 1 serving
Raw nuts: 2 servings
NO dairy products, NO grains, NO junk food, NO added sugar, and NO artificial sweeteners during this phase

Select foods within these categories to meet your daily food plan requirements:

Animal & Seafood Protein
Serving Size 3-4 ounces

Anchovy	Goose	Pork
Bass	Grouper	Quail
Beef (Grass Fed)	Halibut	Salmon
Buffalo (bison)	Herring	Sardines
Catfish	Lamb	Scallops
Chicken	Liver	Shrimp
Chicken Sausage	Lobster	Snapper
Clams	Mackerel	Trout
Cod	Mahi-Mahi	Tuna
Cornish Hen	Mussels	Turkey
Crab	Orange	Turkey Sausage
Duck	Roughy	Venison
Eggs (2 eggs)	Perch	Whitefish
Flounder	Pheasant	

Vegetarian Protein
Serving Size ½ cup cooked

Black Beans	Pinto Beans
Chick Peas	Roman Beans
Garbanzo Beans	Soybeans*
Great Northern Beans	Split Peas
Kidney Beans	White Beans
Lentils	Yellow Beans
Lima Beans	
Navy Beans	

*Limit soybeans to one serving daily

Vegetables - Enjoy fresh or frozen vegetables.
If canned pick options without any added ingredients.

Artichokes	Cucumber	Okra
Arugula	Daikon	Onion
Asparagus	Eggplant	Peas
Bamboo shoots	Endive	Peppers, green
Beans, Green	Fennel	Peppers, red
Bok Choy	Kale	Peppers, yellow
Broccoli	Kohlrabi	Radicchio
Broccoflower	Lettuce, Bibb	Scallions
Brussels Sprouts	Lettuce, Red	Shallots
Cabbage	Leaf	Spinach
Carrots	Lettuce,	Swiss Chard
Cauliflower	Romaine	Tomato
Celery	Lettuce, Bostor	Turnips
Collard Greens	Mushrooms	Water Chestnuts

Fruits – Fresh fruit only, not canned.

Apples	Grapefruit	Pears
Apricots	Grapes	Pineapple
Bananas	Guava	Plantains
Blackberries	Honeydew	Plums
Blueberries	Kiwi	Pomegranates
Boysenberries	Kumquats	Prunes
Cantaloupe	Lemons	Raspberries
Cherries	Limes	Rhubarb
Clementines	Mangos	Starfruit
Coconut	Nectarines	Strawberries
Cranberries	Oranges	Tangerines
Currants	Papayas	Watermelon
Figs	Persimmons	
Gooseberries	Peaches	

Nuts & Seeds   (Serving Size: 1 ounce)
Choose all natural nut butters & nuts/seeds which
do not contain added oils. Look for "raw" or "natural."

Almonds	Peanut butter
Almond Butter	Pecans
Almond Milk	Pine nuts
Cashews	Pumpkin seeds
Chestnuts	Sunflower seeds
Macadamia nuts	Walnuts
Peanuts	

Fats (Serving size =1 tbsp)
Oils should be *cold pressed*

Avocado (1 medium)	Ex. Virgin Olive Oil
Butter	Palm Oil
Coconut Oil	

Station 1 – Reset Your Metabolism

Follow the Metabolic Reset Program exactly for two weeks. It is designed to challenge those habits that you thought you'd never be able to break as well as teach you how to decrease your hunger cravings. It is most effective if the program is performed exactly, without compromise.

The first step of this program, The Metabolic Reset Program, is in essence a detox plan. Most Americans eat processed, sweetened foods at almost every meal. The daily consumption of these foods hijacks your metabolism, bringing it to a grinding halt. These foods also drive your thermostat's set point higher, increasing your hunger and slowing your metabolism. Processed foods also work to sabotage your willpower by increasing your hunger and cravings for toxic food. These toxic food cravings are what drive potato chip and soda pop sales, fill the lines of drive-through-windows across the country, and pack the seats at "family" restaurants that specialize in high-calorie, sweetened, and salted foods at a reasonable price. The most effective way to eliminate these toxic cravings is to address them as what they are – an addiction. Our biologic response to these foods is very similar to what happens after we use tobacco, alcohol, or drugs. The same centers of the brain are triggered and the same needs for larger "doses" with prolonged use are developed.

Slow, Gradual Change

The Metabolic Reset Program represents a perfect *Pound of Cure* diet. At the end of the two weeks, many patients wish to continue with this program because of the amount of weight loss as well as the ability to eat heartily at any time of the day without suffering from the emotional ups and downs and hunger cravings that their previous diet caused. In my practice, I almost always discourage patients from continuing The Metabolic Reset Program for more than two weeks. Eating as described in The Metabolic Reset Program represents a drastic change from most people's current lifestyle. I'm always concerned by extreme and sudden changes in eating habits and typically discourage it in my patients for fear that they are approaching the *Pound of Cure* in the same way they've approached other diet programs.

The approach that I recommend to my patients is a slow, gradual change in your lifestyle. If you follow The Metabolic Reset Program for two weeks, you will eliminate the majority of your cravings for processed food and will be in a position to make good food choices as you move through the remainder of the 12 Stations. By slowly changing your eating behaviors over time in a methodical and meaningful way, you will develop the eating habits that are necessary to not only lose the weight but also nudge your metabolic thermostat downward so that your weight loss is maintained.

It's very common for many people to develop listlessness, difficulty paying attention, and headaches during the first 3-5 days of the diet. These symptoms are not a result of the diet. They are symptoms of withdrawal from the processed foods that you've been eating daily. After these first few days, you'll feel more comfortable and notice that food cravings now seem more manageable. Toward the end of the second week you'll begin to notice that you have more energy, are sleeping better, are in a better mood, and your urges for processed foods and sweets have decreased significantly.

It's important to learn to distinguish between your toxic food cravings and real hunger. Toxic food cravings are characterized by a desire or obsession for a single food, while real hunger produces a desire for any food – the healthier the better. Toxic food cravings often cause headaches, fatigue, nausea, and weakness while true hunger rarely causes any of these symptoms. Toxic food cravings cause gurgling, cramping, and rumbling of your mid and lower abdomen. Many people think that when your "stomach growls" or makes sounds that it is an indication of hunger. This is absolutely not the case. In fact, the air in the intestines makes those sounds and the peristalsis (or movement) of the intestines increases the more toxic the food it contains. Since your stomach lies predominantly underneath your breast bone and in the upper most part of your abdomen, true hunger sensations are typically felt in your lower chest and upper abdomen, not the mid and lower abdomen as most of us have always believed. Finally, true hunger is associated with increased salivation and a heightened taste sensation. When you are really hungry, food tastes absolutely delicious – as the French say, "Hunger makes the best sauce."

It's critically important to recognize the difference between true hunger and toxic food cravings because they need to be addressed separately. True hunger is triggered by your body's thermostat, either as a result of your weight dropping lower than your set point or by your set point being reset to a higher level. Controlling true hunger depends on preventing starvation and eating foods that lower your thermostat. Toxic food cravings are the result of an addiction to the pleasurable brain signals that are triggered by sugar, fat, and whatever additional addictive substances are added to processed food. Controlling toxic food cravings depends on treating the processed food as a substance that you are addicted to, and either cutting down drastically or, better yet, eliminating it completely from your diet.

After a few days on The Metabolic Reset Program, your toxic food cravings should diminish, allowing you to experience predominantly true hunger. Toward the end of the two weeks on the program, you may also notice a reduction in your true hunger as your set point starts its journey downward. Pay attention to the different sensations you experience during the latter part of these two weeks and learn to recognize the difference between true hunger and toxic food cravings.

Challenge Your Daily Habits

Many people find that one or more of their daily habits are directly challenged by the strict guidelines of The Metabolic Reset Program. Many people often make the changes recommended by this program, but ignore one or two of their daily habits, believing that they just can't get by without their morning coffee with cream and sugar or their afternoon diet soda. They believe that as long as they change the other parts of their lives, these daily behaviors won't interfere with their weight loss success. Exactly the opposite is the case! It is your daily habits that require the most scrutiny and should never compromise the rules of the program – because you do them every day! If you have 2 cups of coffee a day and add cream and sugar to each cup, this amounts to over 700 servings of cream and sugar every year. Just the processed food that you add to your morning coffee is enough to raise your thermostat's set point a little bit each year. It is entirely possible that your seemingly innocent daily habits are the reason that you've been unable to lose weight in the past.

The most common habit that is challenged is the regular use of artificially sweetened drinks. A perceived dependence on diet soda, sports drinks, and artificially sweetened creamers in your morning coffee run in direct opposition to the requirements of this station. It is critical that you don't adjust the guidelines to your habits, but rather adjust your habits to the guidelines. Commit to eliminating the artificially sweetened (or full sugar) drinks that you've become dependent on during the two weeks of this station. By the end of the two weeks you'll recognize that these very things that you thought you could never do without were much easier to give up than you ever imagined. It's very likely that these foods were contributing to the difficulty of maintaining your weight, even though they were sugar-free, low carb or fat free, and advertised and touted as weight loss foods.

If you regularly consume diet or regular soda, or sweetened iced teas and don't consume other caffeinated beverages, it can be very difficult to give up these drinks. It's not the soda or tea that is so addictive - it's the caffeine. Caffeine addictions can be very strong and can cause withdrawal symptoms for months. If your only source of caffeine comes from soft drinks or other sweetened beverages, you should add black coffee, green or black tea, or even caffeinated water to ensure that you don't suffer from caffeine withdrawal. With the strategic continuation of your daily caffeine, you'll find that giving up the soda is one of the easier changes that you'll make as you progress through the 12 Stations.

The Metabolic Reset Program

The Metabolic Reset Program focuses on the healthiest foods available and encourages you to eat as much of them as you like. The program allows for three servings of protein for women and four servings of protein for men, daily. The protein can come from either plants (beans) or animals (meat, poultry, or fish). However, at least one of your daily servings must come from the vegetable list. If you are a vegetarian, or would like to become one, you can choose all of your protein servings from the vegetable protein list. If you are not a vegetarian and can never see yourself becoming one, this is fine as well. Just make sure to get at least one vegetable protein serving daily.

The next item on the program is the most critical one. It instructs you to eat at least one pound of vegetables, daily. To reiterate – you must eat **at least** one pound, but one and a half pounds or even two pounds daily is better. These vegetables do not have to be eaten raw, nor do they have to be fresh. Frozen and even canned (assuming no added salt) vegetables are encouraged since they are typically less expensive and do not require the frequent shopping trips that fresh vegetables do.

Fruit is also unlimited during this and every other phase of the program. However, they cannot be dried or canned. It is also **not** necessary to purchase organic fruits, or avoid higher sugar fruits like bananas.

A small amount of fat intake is acceptable but limited to one tablespoon daily. I find it is most useful to place the tablespoon of oil into a BPA-free spritz bottle (that can be purchased at most drug stores) and use it throughout the day to flavor salads or roast vegetables. The acceptable choices for oil are listed and thankfully include both butter and olive oil – the two most common fats used for cooking in most peoples' homes.

Two ounces of nuts and seeds each day is encouraged, though the nuts must be in raw or natural form - not roasted or salted. Raw nuts make an excellent snack and are a powerful appetite suppressant. They also appear to have powerful thermostat lowering properties. Most people eat them in the afternoon and find that helps keep them satisfied until dinnertime.

Finally, the program encourages you to drink lots of water to help flush the processed food toxins out. Dairy products, grains (breads, pastas, oatmeal, etc.), added sugar, and artificial sweeteners are all forbidden on The Metabolic Reset Program. Eliminating these foods ensures that you are eating a diet completely free of processed foods, allowing you to begin to rid yourself of your addictions so you can make good food choices going forward.

It's Easier than You Think

Although many people feel overwhelmed when they review The Metabolic Reset Program, they find out it is much easier to follow than they initially thought. A typical day on the program provides you with more than enough food to ensure that you are never hungry.

Rapid weight loss is very common while you are on The Metabolic Reset Program. In the significantly obese

(>75 pounds overweight), it is common to see patients lose one pound a day for the entire two weeks. While those with less significant obesity typically lose 5-10 pounds over the two weeks.

Once you've completed at least two weeks on The Metabolic Reset Program, and have stuck to it faithfully, you're ready to proceed with the rest of the program. If you are unable to complete two weeks on the program, then it is time to question your commitment to change and willingness to give up those foods that you have convinced yourself you cannot do without. If you are able to follow it faithfully, you will find yourself in the proper state to make good decisions about food. And, you will have learned a lot about the powerful effect of fruits and vegetables and the dangers of grains, dairy, sugar, salt, and artificial sweeteners on your weight.

Breakfast: coffee with almond milk, two pieces of fruit, two-egg omelet with vegetables

Snack: 1 apple, green beans

Lunch: Large salad with black beans, salsa

Snack: 2 ounces of nuts

Dinner: Large plate of roasted broccoli with 4 oz. of Salmon, side of asparagus

Dessert: Two pieces of Fruit

A typical day on the Metabolic Reset Program

Summary

- The Metabolic Reset Program represents a perfect version of the *Pound of Cure* diet.
- You should only stay on the Metabolic Reset Program for two weeks.
- Expect to experience a shortened attention span, mild headaches, and fatigue for the first few days on the program as you detox from processed foods.
- Make sure you adjust your habits to the guidelines, not the guidelines to your habits.
- Toxic food cravings are the result of an addiction to processed food and should be addressed as such.
- True hunger is driven by your metabolic thermostat and should be addressed by eating foods that lower your set point.

Station 2 – One Pound of Vegetables

Eat at least one pound of vegetables daily with your goal being two pounds a day. Limit canned vegetables to those that do not contain added salt. Do not eat the vegetables with any oily or creamy salad dressings or dips.

If the healing properties of a diet that is rich in fruits and vegetables could be captured and placed inside a pill, the resulting medication would be touted the world over as a miracle drug. This drug would be able to rightfully claim to reduce the risk of dozens of types of cancers, improve diabetes, lower blood pressure, and prevent heart disease. Unfortunately, this pill does not exist and likely will not be discovered in our lifetime.

There are so many different micronutrient compounds present in fruits and vegetables that a pill or supplement that contains only a single one is unlikely to make a significant impact on our health. Also, there is a synergistic effect in which the many different compounds mixed together are needed for the health benefits and any one alone has little effect. It is the high density of micronutrients that make vegetables the most powerful thermostat lowering foods on the planet. Intuitively, we all know that increasing the amount of vegetables in our diet results in weight loss, not weight gain.

This station calls for you to eat one pound of vegetables daily to make sure that your body receives plenty of valuable micronutrients. Although one pound of vegetables may initially sound like a large amount, it's actually very manageable. It's likely that you'll be able to easily exceed the one pound mark after a month or so. One 14" cucumber weighs approximately one pound, as do four medium sized tomatoes. Alternatively, six carrots, a small head of celery or 2/3 of a head of broccoli will allow you to meet your one pound goal. In fact, it's very reasonable to eat one pound of vegetables in a single sitting – my lunchtime salad in the hospital cafeteria always exceeds one pound.

Micronutrients

Although meats, fish, and poultry are rich in vitamins and minerals, they typically do not contain many of the life extending anti-oxidant micronutrients that play a critical role in our health by preventing chronic diseases. There are tens of thousands of these different compounds - they include lycopenes (found in tomatoes and other red colored fruits and vegetables), bioflavonoids (found in citrus, tea, wine and dark chocolate), resveratrol (found in chocolate, grapes, peanuts and wine), sulforaphane (found in broccoli and Brussels sprouts), and countless others that have yet to be discovered. They are present in the largest amounts in vegetables with fruits and nuts containing slightly lower amounts and little being found in grains. They are typically not found in meat, fish or poultry. There is ample evidence in medical literature that demonstrates that a micronutrient rich diet of fruits and vegetables is protective against Alzheimer's dementia, diabetes, heart disease, many cancers, and obesity.

It is likely that these anti-oxidant compounds play an important role in driving down our metabolic thermostat to a lower weight. The impact of vegetables is cumulative over time. The more vegetables you eat each day, and the longer you've been eating them, the lower your thermostat's set point will drop. Many patients find, that after a year of eating one and a half or two pounds of vegetables daily, they are much more resistant to the weight gain effects of processed food. The inevitable moments that you stray from your *Pound of Cure* eating style will not result in the rapid weight regain that typically occurs after breaking a starvation diet.

This station aims to get you used to eating vegetables, both raw and cooked in large quantities, without oily or creamy dressings or dips. There are no other restrictions to this station of the program other than eating mindfully and doing your best to avoid unhealthy foods. It is very likely that your increased vegetable intake will decrease your cravings for less healthy foods. I also encourage you to vary the type of vegetables you eat and expand your horizons beyond the popular staples of broccoli, carrots, and tomatoes.

Green Leafy Vegetables

Without a doubt, the most nutritious foods on the planet are green, leafy vegetables: specifically spinach, leaf lettuces, romaine lettuce, kales, greens, cabbage, bok-choy, and parsley (notice the absence of iceberg lettuce from this list). I urge you to explore these leafy green vegetables and get used to eating them several times a day. They often come pre-cleaned and cut up and are relatively inexpensive making them convenient snacks and side dishes. In my practice, I often refer to the 100 calorie snack pack of spinach to emphasize how nutrient dense green leafy vegetables are. The standard one-pound bag of spinach contains around 100 calories. Compare it to the 100-calorie snack pack of cookies which usually weigh less than one ounce.

Other green vegetables like broccoli, asparagus, Brussels sprouts, cucumbers, green peppers, peas, string beans, and celery are also excellent choices. These vegetables can be eaten either raw or cooked. Frozen vegetables contain almost the same nutritional value as fresh vegetables and make excellent choices. Canned vegetables often have added salt and you should limit your intake to low-salt varieties. Vegetable soups are also excellent choices. Other vegetables like mushrooms, onions, tomatoes, yellow and red peppers, cauliflower, carrots, beets, and eggplants are extremely dense in the nutrients that will drive down your metabolic thermostat. Finally, beans and legumes have the added benefit of containing large amounts of protein making them particularly important to your diet. Dry beans need to be soaked before cooking which requires advanced planning. Canned beans are much more convenient and typically don't have large amounts of added salt.

Plan for Success

Initially, ensuring that you consume a pound of vegetables daily will require some planning. You may need to cut them up in advance and pack them in individual baggies to be eaten throughout the day. Over time, you will find that vegetables satisfy many of your cravings for crunchy snack foods and significantly decrease your appetite during mealtime causing you to eat less at each sitting than you used to. Ultimately, you will find yourself gravitating toward vegetables and find the one pound requirement is an easy mark that you will exceed without difficulty.

There is a dose effect for vegetables – if one pound is good, two pounds is better. Vegetables are unique. Contrary to every other food group, the more vegetables you eat, the more weight you will lose. Eating one pound of vegetables a day will change your eating habits significantly; however the real magic occurs when you reach the two pound mark. If you regularly eat two pounds of vegetables daily, you will find that your desire for fattening processed foods will disappear as your metabolic thermostat drops. At two pounds daily, your weight loss will accelerate with many patients losing 8-10 pounds per month while eating a larger volume of food than ever before. Again, because of the effects of the vegetables on your metabolic thermostat, your metabolism will increase and your hunger will decrease as the pounds melt away.

Vegetables as the Centerpiece of the Meal

Most Americans make the protein component of a meal the main focus. When asked what you ate for dinner last night, most of us will reply with "chicken," "fish," or "beef" without commenting on the vegetables. This is because the primary focus is the protein. The vegetables and other side dishes are viewed as secondary in importance. This eating plan aims to change that, making the vegetables the primary focus and the protein the flavor enhancer. For instance, a large plate of Brussels sprouts mixed with a few pieces of crushed turkey bacon ensures that you eat primarily vegetables for dinner, but still get the flavor of the protein in every bite. In essence, every meal should be a salad with the majority of the food on your plate consisting of vegetables while the more fattening animal proteins, nuts and seeds, constitute an ingredient used to add flavor to the dish.

It's not necessary to eat a salad, in the conventional sense, at every meal in order to satisfy the requirements of this station. As you get used to this eating style, you'll come up with your own way to honor your goal of making the vegetables the largest portion of any meal. For instance, rather than the typical 8-10 oz. piece of salmon that most Americans eat for dinner, you'll find that a 3-4 oz. piece served on top of a large plate of lightly roasted Bok-choy can be equally satisfying for dinner. By chopping the salmon and mixing it in with the Bok-choy, every bite will contain the salmon flavor. You'll leave the table feeling more satisfied because you ate 2-3 times more food than if you had eaten a larger piece of salmon.

Another strategy to increase your vegetable intake and reduce the amount of grain and animal proteins in your diet is to replace the grain component of a meal with a green leafy vegetable and cut back on the animal proteins. One of my favorite foods is hamburgers, but these are obviously not part of the *Pound of Cure* plan. By converting the hamburger sandwich into a salad, it can become a healthy choice that can be eaten heartily. Instead of the bun, add a large amount of leafy greens to a four-ounce grass fed hamburger patty. Then add lots of tomatoes, lightly grilled onions and mushrooms, pickles, ketchup, mustard and even a little bit of avocado. The salad will have all the taste of a hamburger, but will not leave you feeling bloated, uncomfortable, and guilty for straying from the plan.

Salad Dressing

People are often taken aback by the recommendation to eat a salad without any salad dressing. We've been convinced by the food and diet industry that salad dressing is a critical part of the salad - as important as the lettuce. The marketing of low fat and low carb dressings by the diet industry further supports the perception that our vegetables can only be enjoyed if they taste like the rest of processed food – oily, salty, and sweet. Many people find that eating the salad without dressing is a simple adjustment. However, some people never seem to be able to make the change. For those people I recommend using salsa, hummus (no added oil), lemon juice, vinegars (balsamic, red wine, apple cider and other flavors), and nut based dressings located in the recipe section at the back of this book. There is an increasing market for salad dressings without added oils or sugars that use nuts and nut butters as the base with added herbs and spices for flavors. Seek out these nut based dressings. But, read the labels closely since many do contain added oils and sugars. Better yet, make your own from our recipe list or from others found on the Internet.

Set Point Smoothies

If you find yourself stuck at the one pound mark and want to push your intake further, a very effective way to increase this is to start drinking what I refer to as "Set Point Smoothies" every day. Set Point Smoothies are made by blending a green leafy vegetable (spinach, kale, turnip or collard greens, etc.) with a sweet fruit (strawberries, bananas, blueberries, pineapple, etc.), an herb or spice (cilantro, ginger root, etc.), and a little ice or coconut milk. These drinks make an excellent breakfast along with a few pieces of fruit. Also, drinking a Set Point Smoothie before dinner will typically reduce the amount of food you eat when you sit down for your meal. Those of you who suffer from night time hunger can put this to bed with an after dinner Set Point Smoothie. Feel free to adjust this recipe to your own tastes. Most of my patients try these with some initial reluctance, but quickly realize their value in controlling hunger and ensuring that they reach the one pound mark daily. Set Point Smoothies are the closest thing to a portable, palatable supplement that can lower your metabolic thermostat if taken daily – remember this when you take your first sip.

Finding a good grocer to support your pound a day vegetable habit is a critical component to success. Although more and more specialty grocery stores are popping up that contain an excellent produce section, even the best still offer mostly processed foods. Unfortunately, the vegetable industry pales in profitability compared to the vitamin, diet food, dairy, meat, and grain industry. Years ago, before the processed food industry exploded, the vegetable industry played a significant role in the American food chain. Vegetables were even marketed on television (remember the Jolly Green Giant?) Today, the Green Giant Company is owned by General Mills whose sale of frozen vegetables makes up only a small percentage of their total profits. The American food chain consists primarily of processed foods that drive the profits of several multi-billion dollar companies. Long-term success will depend on abandoning the traditional American food chain and opting for unprocessed, unadvertised alternatives from the produce department.

Organics

Many people feel the need to purchase organic produce, worried that the traditional produce is filled with harmful chemicals. While organic produce is healthier than traditional produce, in general the benefits are not warranted by the much higher price. If you desire the healthiest food possible and are not swayed by the increased price, feel free to purchase organic fruits and vegetables. If the price of organic produce is prohibitive, do not feel as if you are compromising your health by opting for traditional produce. For those who wish to take the middle ground, reserve your organic purchases for fruits or vegetables that have thin or no skin: such as apples, grapes, lettuce, peaches and pears.

Many people may seek out their local farmer's markets to obtain low cost, organic produce. Farmer's markets were fairly uncommon a few years ago. Most cities could only support a few markets. Over the last few years, they are on the rise and now most towns contain at least one, if not multiple markets. Unfortunately, many of them do not contain high-quality, inexpensive or organic produce. In fact, some of the stands are not run by farmers. They're run by vendors who purchase the produce, usually from the same distributors as the grocery stores, and inflate the price assuming people will believe that the produce is organic. When shopping at farmer's markets, it's important to ask questions about the farm that grew the produce. Look for farms that raise livestock in addition to growing fruits and vegetables since animals are integral to a sustainable organic farm. Also ask about the types of crops that are grown. If the answer is corn and soybeans, move on to the next stand. Despite the questionable quality of many of the new, smaller, farmer's markets, most cities still have a few stable, high-quality markets that provide you an opportunity to purchase high-quality, organic produce directly from the farmers at a fair price. As you move further along the *Pound of Cure* program, a quality farmer's market will make the job of finding produce at a fair price a little easier.

This station is the most important one of the entire program and will likely take at least a month until the task of eating a pound of vegetables daily develops into a preference for vegetables over other foods. It is only through the copious intake of vegetables that you will be able to reduce your dependency on other, less healthy foods. When you find yourself spending the majority of your shopping trip in the produce section, enjoying giant salads without dressing, and grabbing a handful of raw carrots as a snack, you are ready for the next station.

Summary

- One pound of vegetables is just a minimum — aim for two pounds.

- Vegetables are the most potent thermostat lowering foods; make sure that you have cut vegetables readily available.

- Vegetables should be the centerpiece of every meal.

- Experiment with vinegars, salsa, hummus, and nut based salad dressings.

- Set Point Smoothies represent the closest thing to a supplement that can be used to lower your metabolic thermostat.

- Organic produce is preferable, but not necessary for your success.

Vegetables – A thorough but not complete list

artichokes
arugula
asparagus
bamboo shoot
beans, black
beans, cannellini
beans, garbanzo
beans, great northern
beans, green
beans, kidney
beans, lentil
beans, lima
beans, navy
beans, pinto
beans, roman
beans, white
beans, yellow
beets
bok-choy
Boston lettuce
broccoli

broccoflower
Brussels sprouts
cabbage
carrots
cauliflower
celery
chick peas
collard greens
cucumber
daikon
eggplant
endive
fennel
kale
kohlrabi
mushrooms
okra
onion
parsley
peas, black eyed
peas, green

peas, snap
peas, snow
peas, split
peppers, green
peppers, red
peppers, yellow
radicchio
radishes
red leaf lettuce
romaine lettuce
scallions
shallots
soybeans
spinach
squash
Swiss chard
tomato
turnips
water chestnuts
zucchini

Station 3 – Replace Sweetened Foods with Fruit

Eat at least four servings of fruit per day, but avoid fruit juice and dried fruit. Limit sugar sweetened and artificial sweetened foods to 1-2 servings per week.

America's increased consumption of sugar has directly paralleled our increased rate of obesity, leading many to believe that sugar is the primary cause of our nation's weight problem. A few states are even instituting a sugar tax to increase the cost of high-sugar foods in an effort to deter people from consuming them. The data is becoming clearer every day. Sugar's reputation is well deserved. In fact, it's likely that the dangers of sugar have been underrepresented. Some researchers are insisting that sugar is not just an unhealthy indulgence in our diet, but rather a toxin that is destroying our health. Although we've known for decades that sugar consumption leads to weight gain, evidence is mounting that supports sugar's role in high blood pressure, heart disease, Alzheimer's disease, and even many cancers. One of the most frightening studies demonstrates that many of these changes in your body's chemistry can occur after only a few weeks of a high-sugar diet.

There's been a lot of negative attention directed at high fructose corn syrup; much to the chagrin of the corn industry and the appreciation of the sugar industry. With the attention directed at high fructose corn syrup, sugar has been allowed to slide under the radar; making claims that sugar is natural and that it's the evil corn industry creating high fructose corn syrup that is to blame. Well, it's becoming quite clear – both sugar and high fructose corn syrup are equally bad and both must be avoided.

Sugar

Avoiding sugar is quite difficult, since it's found in so many foods. Ketchup, sushi, pickles, cereals (even the organic ones), fast food, and breads all contain high amounts of either sugar or high fructose corn syrup. It's the ubiquitous nature of sugar that has caused the average American's consumption to increase from 70 grams per day in the 1970's to almost 200 grams today. This near tripling of the amount of sugar consumed is due to the improvements made in refining techniques and the advent of high fructose corn syrup leading to inexpensive, government-subsidized sweeteners. It is now very inexpensive to add sugar to processed food products which explains why it is so hard to avoid eating foods with added sugar.

The continual presence of sugar in our diet has led to many people developing an addiction to sugar. This is not surprising since sugar triggers the pleasure centers of our brain. Over time, it takes higher doses of sugar to trigger the same response, leading to the development of tolerance. This addictive tendency can easily be demonstrated by putting a large, sugary dessert in front of someone and asking them to eat just one bite. It takes an incredible amount of will power to have just one bite - much more so than for other foods.

This same effect has been demonstrated in animal studies. If rats are given both a sugared drink and food they will gradually increase their intake of the sugared drink over time until it consists of the majority of their caloric intake. Humans have the tendency to do the same if given the opportunity.

Soft Drinks

Regular soft drink consumption is perhaps the most dangerous way to ingest sugar. Soft drinks contain staggering amounts of sugar. One 20 oz. Coca Cola contains 65 grams of sugar (that's about 27 sugar cubes). Energy drinks, iced teas, lemonades, and fruit juices are not much better, containing, on average only 10% less sugar than Coca Cola. The clear link between soft drinks (both carbonated and non-carbonated) and childhood obesity has caused some states to ban soda and sweetened milk drinks in public schools. Additionally, most soda contains large amounts of sodium. The salty taste is covered up by the sugar. Salt will act to stimulate your thirst, driving you to drink more. Because of the salt, sugar and caffeine in soda, it is as addictive as tobacco - and perhaps even more detrimental to your health.

Soda is the only food that has been statistically linked to obesity. I believe that soft drinks are the most powerful thermostat raising foods on the planet and should be eliminated from the diet of anyone seeking to lose weight or improve their health. The thermostat raising effects of sugar sweetened sodas are almost immediate. There is a bounty of evidence that demonstrates that liquid calorie intake will cause an immediate imbalance between the consumption and expenditure of calories. Sugary drinks work in the same way that corticosteroids and other medications that cause weight gain do. These drinks immediately shift your thermostat higher, resulting in increased hunger and calorie consumption without an equal amount of calorie expenditure. The net result is - of course - weight gain. Solid sweetened foods like cookies and cakes can have a similar but much less pronounced effect. Naturally sweetened foods that contain fiber like fruits and some vegetables do not appear to have any thermostat raising effects, and for this reason, are critical components of the *Pound of Cure* program.

Fruit

Many people are very quick to claim that fruit also contains sugar and is therefore nearly as bad as cookies, cupcakes, and soda. Although the critics of a diet rich in fruits are correct that fruit contains sugar, their argument that fruit results in weight gain is off the mark.

When eating sweetened, processed foods, sugar is rapidly absorbed into the bloodstream and the sugar is shipped directly to the liver, causing immediate storage as fat. Further, sugar has the unique ability to block the release of leptin, a very strong inhibitor of our appetite. Since the sugar fails to trigger leptin release, your hunger drive does not shut down, causing you to eat more. Leptin is one of the primary mechanisms that your metabolic thermostat uses to shut down your hunger in response to reaching the overfed state. By poisoning this critical pathway, your metabolic thermostat is allowed to inch upward by a very small amount. If this process is repeated several times a day, the net result can be a significant upward shift in your thermostat's setting.

When sugar is eaten in the form of fruit, the fiber in the fruit will slow the absorption of sugar (not block it completely) resulting in less of the sugar being converted to fat. More importantly, the fiber in the fruit triggers the release of leptin, effectively canceling out the inhibitory effect of the sugar. In short, nature packages both the poison and the antidote together, allowing fruit to be eaten liberally without altering your thermostat's set point.

If you want to consume as much sugar as the average American eats daily (200 grams) solely in the form of fruit, you better bring your appetite; you'll need to eat around 15 pieces of fruit. Most decadent desserts (a half pint of ice cream, apple pie a la mode, or a big piece of chocolate cake) contain over 150 grams of sugar on their own and do little to impact your appetite.

You should feel free to eat as many servings of fruit as you wish without fear that it contains too many calories or too much sugar. Fruit is your best weapon against your sweet cravings and should be employed maximally. Holding back on fruit leaves you open to an attack from that break room doughnut. Try to eat at least four servings of fruit per day, but avoid fruit juice and dried fruit since these are too calorie dense to make them good choices. Additionally, fruit juice and dried fruit do not help to control your appetite the way raw fruit does. Fruit smoothies that do not contain vegetables should be limited since they allow for you to ingest them quickly before you begin to feel full. The Set Point Smoothies discussed in the last station can be consumed without limits.

Artificial Sweeteners

America has a long history of trying to minimize sugar consumption. For decades, sugar free was equated with guilt free. Eating and drinking sugar free foods allowed us to continue our indulgences and predilection for sweetness without having to worry about its effect on our waistline. We're now starting to learn that artificially sweetened foods often cause as many problems as the sugar it's replacing and likely fan the flames of our powerful addiction to sweets.

The first artificial sweetener, saccharin, was developed in 1879 at Johns Hopkins. It became popular during World War II when a sugar shortage forced housewives to use it as an alternative to sugar. Since saccharin, many other sweeteners have been discovered: including aspartame (Nutrasweet®), Acesulfame Potassium (acesulfame K®), Sucralose (Splenda®), and most recently Stevia (Truvia®). Although most people associate these sweeteners with the pink, blue, yellow, and green packets they add to their morning coffee, their greatest consumption occurs from their inclusion in consumer foods and beverages. These products are included in nearly every "diet," "light," and "low-carb" product on the market resulting in many people consuming 3-5 servings per day. Even most protein shakes that are recommended in many weight loss regimens are artificially sweetened.

In the 1970's when artificial sweeteners were first beginning to become popular, there were some reports that saccharin (Sweet & Low®) caused bladder cancer in male rats. Due to these reports, the USDA attempted to completely ban saccharin in 1972. Subsequent studies questioned the validity of the initial reports and it is now believed that saccharin does not increase your risk of developing cancer. Similar accusations were originally levied against Nutrasweet®, claiming that it increased your risk of developing brain cancer, however these claims were never proven. To date, there is no conclusive evidence that any of the artificial sweeteners on the market increase your risk of developing cancer.

Although there is little evidence directly linking artificial sweeteners to specific medical conditions, there is a significant amount of evidence linking diet soft drinks to vascular disease, diabetes, heart disease, high blood pressure, and high cholesterol. Most of the impact was seen in those individuals who drank multiple diet soft drinks daily. It remains unclear whether or not it is the artificial sweeteners or the other chemicals in the soft drink that are responsible for the negative effects.

There is growing evidence that demonstrates that eating artificially sweetened foods leads to obesity. Now that we understand that an upward shift in our metabolic thermostat causes weight gain (not an excess of calories), the negative impact of calorie free foods on our weight seems more plausible. It appears that artificial sweeteners' ability to trigger the sweet sensors in your brain may also shift your thermostat's set point higher. Their impact on your thermostat triggers an increase in your hunger while slowing your metabolic rate. Despite the lack of calories, artificially sweetened foods can cause weight gain.

Addicted to Sweet

Our body's response to a sweet taste is a powerful evolutionary advantage. Because no natural foods on this planet that contains fructose are poisonous, the sweet taste that fructose triggers is a guarantee that the food we are eating is safe. Because of this phenomenon, our body is hard wired to seek out sweet-tasting food to ensure that we don't starve. When we get our hands on anything sweet our brain triggers an "eat up – it's safe" signal, driving us to eat more.

There are many studies that demonstrate that sugar stimulates the pleasure centers of the brain. This triggering drives us to eat more and eventually we can develop addictions to sweet tastes just as we can to drugs, alcohol, and cigarettes. Although artificial sweeteners are not the same as sugar, they trigger the same taste receptors and reward centers in our brain, continually strengthening our addiction even if we're eating very little sugar. The same effect is found when treating a heroin addict with the drug methadone.

Methadone is a long-acting, less powerful version of heroin that can be taken in pill form. Regular intake of methadone can help a heroin addict refrain from injecting the drug for years, but does nothing to break the addiction. Some argue that a heroin addict who uses methadone has a stronger craving for the drug than one who uses heroin regularly. The same argument may be made for the regular users of artificially sweetened foods in relation to their addiction to sugar.

Taste Adaptation

Another way that artificially sweetened foods are dangerous to our health is because of a process known as "taste adaptation." Artificial sweeteners are 200-7,000 times sweeter than sugar. This much more intense sweetness can trigger our taste receptors to their maximal response resulting in our development of tolerance for sweet tastes. Regular use of artificial sweeteners requires more and more of the sweet taste to trigger the pleasure centers in our brain. This causes our intake of artificially sweetened food to escalate. As a related bystander, our intake of sugar typically does as well. Even worse, regular use of artificial sweeteners and sugar causes healthy sweetened food, like fruit, to fall flat on our palate, making fruit appear bland and tasteless by comparison. Just like all addictive substances, abstaining from sugar and artificially sweetened foods and drinks will result in a normalization of our taste receptors and our brain's desire for sweetness.

Stevia is a "natural" sweetener that does not contain calories and has been touted as the "safe" alternative to sugar. It is an extract made from the stevia plant and is 200-300 times sweeter than sugar. Again, the intense sweetness of Stevia results in taste adaptations that drive your cravings for sugar and artificially sweetened foods. Also, Stevia is an extract, not a whole, natural food and is not a better choice than any of the other artificial sweeteners. Keep in mind that sugar is an extract of many natural foods like sugar cane and beets, but this does not make it a healthy choice. Stevia, like the other sweeteners should be avoided.

Despite the widespread popularity of artificial sweeteners, our addiction to sugar remains strong. The average American eats just shy of 200 grams (1/2 a cup) of either sugar or high fructose corn syrup daily. Our consumption of artificial sweeteners is similarly impressive. In order to break free of our addiction to sweetness, it is critical to provide our bodies with plenty of fruit and avoid sugar and sugar substitutes as much as possible. Once free of the sugar, we can derive nearly the same enjoyment from fruit without the weight gain and negative health consequences.

Summary

- Sugar is addictive and will prevent you from losing weight.
- Soft drinks are the most thermostat raising of all foods – even diet sodas cause weight gain.
- Fruit is nutrient dense and can be eaten in unlimited amounts.
- Use fruit to satisfy your sweet cravings.
- Artificial sweeteners contribute to weight gain by raising your thermostat's set point. Avoid them.

Station 4 – Move Your Body

Wear a pedometer every day and increase the number of steps you take each day by 50%. Resolve to take the stairs as much as possible, aiming for 10 flights up a day.

The primary goal of this station is to increase your daily physical activity by 50%. Although physical activity is not an important part of weight loss, it is critical for good health. Yes, you read that correctly – physical activity is not a particularly important component of a weight loss program. This does not mean that I don't recommend increasing your physical activity and exercising. It is critical for **maintaining** your weight loss and it's absolutely mandatory for good health. In my practice, one of the most common reasons for weight loss failure is over-relying on exercise for weight loss and not paying enough attention to food choices.

It's important to distinguish physical activity from exercise. Physical activity is the amount of movement that you perform throughout the entire day whereas exercise is extreme physical activity performed for a short period of time. In short, physical activity does not require a change of clothes, exercise does.

As we discussed earlier, building healthy muscle can help to shift your thermostat's set point downward - facilitating weight loss. All thermostat raising or lowering

49

factors have varying degrees of success from person to person. Bariatric surgery can cause some people to effortlessly shrink down to a size 2 while others lose much less weight. Medications and diet changes also have variable effects across individuals. I've found that there is a tremendous variation in the impact of physical activity and exercise on weight loss. A few patients find that a walking program or exercise regimen are extremely helpful and cause a rapid and effortless weight loss. Most find that it has little impact. Nonetheless, increasing your walking and stair climbing can help to shift your thermostat downward and it is important that we thoroughly explore all tools at our disposal. Research evaluating the behaviors present in individuals who are able to lose weight and keep it off demonstrates that regular walking and exercise activities help more with weight maintenance than with weight loss. This implies that at the very least, increased physical activity acts as a stabilizing agent for your thermostat's set point, ensuring that it does not creep back up after you've worked so hard to lower it.

This station focuses on increasing physical activity, not on starting an exercise program. No matter how much or how little daily activity you perform on average, we can always increase it by making a few small adjustments to your lifestyle.

Pedometers

The best way to ensure that you are increasing your physical activity is to wear a pedometer. A pedometer is a small device that you wear on your belt, as a watch, or carry in your pocket that measures the number of steps you take throughout the day. They range in price from $5 to $150. The features and accuracy vary as well. Although the extra features can be fun, they are not necessary for you to complete this station. A simple pedometer that just measures the total number of steps will suffice. Before you get started, I recommend experimenting with the device to make sure that it's accurate. You may have to change where you wear it on your body. Also, make sure to select a pedometer with the reset button properly shielded so that you don't hit it accidentally and erase the total number of steps you have taken throughout the day.

After you have the pedometer working appropriately, wear it for a few days to determine what your baseline physical activity is. It's important to get an average over a few days rather than to use the measurement from your first day. The goal for this station is to increase the number of steps you take every day by 50% (i.e. if you are taking 5,000 steps per day, you want to increase by 50%, or 2,500 steps for a total of 7,500 steps per day). It is not necessary to make this increase overnight. It's better to increase by 10% per week, taking five weeks to work yourself up to your new level of activity. Get in the habit of wearing the pedometer every day and adjusting your activity to ensure you reach your goal. Don't stop wearing the pedometer after you have moved on to the next station. Take the pedometer off for any planned exercise sessions during the day. The goal is just to increase your daily physical activity and not to make modifications to your exercise program – this will come later.

Here is a breakdown of how the number of steps that you take each day correlates with your level of activity:

Number of Steps per Day	Activity Level
<100	Immobile
100-999	Disabled
1,000 – 3,000	Sedentary
4,000 – 7,000	Average
7,000 – 10,000	Active
>10,000	Athletic

There are countless ways to increase the number of steps that you take each day. The simplest is to go for a walk – one mile is usually around 2,000 steps. Although you can simply add in a 1-2 mile walk every day to reach your goal, this technique leaves you susceptible to the weather and your work and home responsibilities to ensure that it is completed each day. To reliably reach your new goal, you will have to adjust the way you look at your daily routine. Consider the following possibilities:

- Unless the weather prohibits, look for the worst possible parking space you can find. Rather than making your parking goal to find a spot as close to the store as possible, try to park as far away as possible. You'll never have any difficulty getting a spot and won't risk the fender benders that inevitably will occur if you circle a busy parking lot enough times.
- If you have any regular meetings, offer to have a walking meeting where you discuss business while walking, rather than sitting down. One of the greatest entrepreneurs of the modern era, Steve Jobs, was well known for his walking meetings.
- If you work at a desk, consider a treadmill desk. These desks allow you to work while walking at a slow pace on a treadmill, rather than sitting in a chair. These things are not a gimmick – it's possible to be productive and increase your physical activity at the same time. Most people who switch to a treadmill desk report a 200-300% increase in their daily pedometer readouts.
- If you regularly walk the dog, double the distance of the walk. Make it your new routine – your dog will love you for it.

- Go to an indoor mall and window shop for an hour.
- Garden, shovel snow, or clean your house every day.
- Disconnect your cable for the summer.
- Go for a family walk after dinner.

There are many other ways that you can increase the number of steps you take each day and you are the best person to figure out how to change your routine. This station, like the others, is about changing your daily habits in small, meaningful ways, over time. The pedometer holds the key to ensuring that you are meeting your goal and more importantly, maintaining this goal. Plan to continue to wear it long after you move past this station.

Climbing Stairs

Beyond increasing the number of steps that you take every day, commit to taking the stairs as much as possible with your goal being more than 10 flights up a day. Some of the more expensive pedometers will measure the number of flights of stairs that you walk up each day. The stairwell can serve as an inexpensive, convenient, exercise machine that should be installed in your daily routine. Even more so than walking, stairs are an excellent measure of your overall health and fitness. The number of flights that you can walk up is one of the most important determinants of your functional status.

Use it or Lose it

Failure to continually work and develop your functional status - your ability to actively participate in life - will lead to its rapid decline. Paralysis or temporary injuries used to be the most common cause of confinement to a wheelchair in adults. Today it is a loss of functional status. When I see patients in my practice with limited mobility and require a cane, walker, or wheelchair to move around, they almost always report that their disability is the result of an orthopedic injury. However, further questioning reveals that it is the result of a slow and gradual deterioration of their joints and muscle strength that started after an injury. A prolonged period of inactivity results in a loss of healthy muscle and therefore an upward shift in your thermostat's set point. The associated weight gain is worsened by your limited ability to burn calories as a result of limited mobility. Often, injuries can cause a frustrating cycle of weight gain that worsens the stress on the injured joint or muscle, causing the accumulation of additional excess weight which slows or prevents recovery.

Because of the difficulty of escaping this cycle and its often permanent effect on your body weight, it is critical that you continually work to improve your functional status. Functional status is a spectrum, with the most fit being able to climb 20 flights of stairs, or more, without stopping. The average, healthy adult is able to climb 4-5 flights without stopping and the inactive person is limited to one flight or even less before needing to stop. A loss of functional status is not caused by a rapid drop from one end of the spectrum to the other, but rather a slow, gradual loss of function until simply walking becomes challenging. In order to ensure that you remain functional well into your senior years, work to keep your functional status at the high end of the spectrum. This will ensure that you have an adequate cushion and avoid the slow, gradual decline toward premature disability and weight gain.

I once overheard a health conscious colleague of mine respond to an inquiry after he emerged from the stairwell on the 8th floor, slightly out of breath. He was asked why he walked up eight flights rather than waiting for the elevator. His response was quite profound - he walked up eight flights of steps "because he can."

Summary

- Increase your daily physical activity levels by walking more and climbing stairs.
- Wear a pedometer to measure your daily steps.
- Walking every day and climbing stairs will improve your functional status and stabilize your metabolic thermostat's set point.
- Aim to improve your functional status to prevent disability.

Station 5 – Raw Nuts, not Roasted

Eat 1-2 ounces of raw nuts daily. Avoid roasted and salted nuts. Also, experiment with raw nut butters as the base of a salad dressing instead of oil.

Nuts are one of the most nutritious foods on the planet. Nuts have high amounts of all three macronutrients (protein, carbohydrates and fat). Nuts tend to be high in fiber as well. Although nuts have lots of calories and have long been considered fattening, there is little evidence that supports this assumption. In fact, we're discovering that just the opposite is true. There are multiple studies that demonstrate that individuals who eat large amounts of nuts daily tend to have lower rates of obesity. This fact is yet another demonstration that the overly simple "calories in verses calories out" theory of weight loss does not hold up. It's likely that nuts serve to lower our thermostat's set point - not raise it.

Nut consumption is also linked to a lower rate of heart disease and diabetes. The daily intake of raw nuts and nut butters will contribute significantly to your appetite control, decreasing your cravings for processed snack foods. There are significantly less health benefits of roasted nuts, and even fewer of roasted, salted nuts.

Nuts – The Preparation Matters

Nuts can be prepared in many different ways and it's the preparation that determines the healthfulness, much more than the type of nut. Here is a breakdown of the healthfulness of different preparation techniques.

Raw (a.k.a. Natural)

Dry Roasted, unsalted

Dry Roasted, Salted

Roasted, Salted

Roasted, Salted, Sweetened

Most Healthy
↓
Least Healthy

Nuts can either be roasted by heating them without any added oils (dry roasted), or heated in the presence of oil (roasted). Frequently, dangerous hydrogenated oils are used in the roasting process, taking a perfectly healthy nut and making it toxic. This is equivalent to deep frying cauliflower or zucchini. Nuts are frequently salted which has two very dangerous effects. The first is that it dramatically increases the sodium content which is bad for your blood pressure. The second is that adding salt to food dramatically increases your appetite and reduces the satiety effects of the food. Raw nuts are very satiating (meaning they make you feel full). The next time you are feeling hungry, eat 1 ounce of raw almonds, cashews, or walnuts and wait ten minutes – your hunger will decrease significantly. Try the same experiment with dry roasted, salted nuts – if anything, you'll feel hungrier.

The dry roasting technique seems harmless enough, but the process of heating nuts can decrease the beneficial health effects significantly and likely makes them more fattening. Raw nuts contain lots of healthy oils. These natural oils are less likely than other oils to contribute to the development of obesity and atherosclerosis of your blood vessels. It's possible that nut oils serve to lower your thermostat, despite their high calorie content.

When you toast nuts, the healthy oils are brought to the surface of the nuts, giving them a richer, oilier taste which we prefer. However, the oils are also transformed. A portion of the natural oils in the nut are converted into a trans-fat. Trans-fats are the least healthy of all oils and are well known to cause obesity. They are very potent thermostat raising agents. There is also a direct correlation between the temperature and duration of the roasting process and the resulting healthfulness of the nuts. If you have trouble enjoying raw nuts, you can lightly toast them for a few minutes at low heat as an alternative to buying them dry roasted. Although you may find raw nuts bland and tasteless at first, in time you will begin to enjoy them as much as their roasted counterparts. Also, as you learn the powerful satiating effects of raw nuts, you can use them as an appetite suppressant that decreases your cravings for dangerous processed foods.

The bottom line for nut preparation techniques are these: eat raw nuts preferentially, or lightly toast them yourself. Avoid salted nuts and nuts roasted in oils. You can also mix raw and roasted nuts 50/50 to enhance the flavor if you can't enjoy raw nuts alone.

All nuts and seeds contain significant health benefits and you should eat a mixture rather than focusing on 1-2 types. Although peanuts are actually legumes not nuts (they come from plants, not trees), they are very healthy and should be treated as nuts from a nutritional perspective. The best way to purchase nuts is in their shell. It's less expensive, and makes it very difficult to over-eat since you'll have to crack each one open.

Nut Based Salad Dressings

Nut based salad dressings are also growing in popularity. Rather than oil as the backbone of the dressing, you can use nut butters. These contain no refined oils or processed food, yet still maintain the creamy taste that we've come to expect from a salad dressing. You can blend raw nuts, flavored vinegar, coconut or almond milk, spices, and onions or garlic into a salad dressing. It tastes great and does not contain the dangerous fats and sugars found in commercial salad dressings. There are several examples of delicious, oil-free salad dressings in the recipe section that should serve as a starting point for your experimentation with these much healthier salad dressings. By making your own dressing, you can also ensure that it contains the healthiest, raw versions of the nuts. Alternatively, you can add nuts or seeds directly to your salad. Also, nut "flours" made of crushed nuts can be used as breading for fish and poultry.

Nut butters are also a great way to expand your diet. Look for 100% natural peanut, cashew, sunflower and almond butters. Nut butters without added salt are ideal, but these can be hard to find and, quite frankly, are a little on the bland side. Eating 100% natural nut butter with a little salt makes a far better choice than a creamy dressing, dip, or processed snack food.

Again, look for nut butters made from raw nuts, not roasted. Avoid most popular commercial nut butters since almost all contain lots of sugar and frequently added oils. Although they are used infrequently, trans-fats are added to low cost nut butters. Make sure to read labels carefully. If a nut butter does not contain added oils, the natural oils in the nuts will separate out and form a layer at the top of the jar. Nut butters that are 100% natural require stirring before use while those with added oils do not. The oil layer at the top of the jar serves as an indicator that the nut butter is 100% natural. Tahini (made from sesame seeds) has similar health benefits but is typically used differently from other nut butters from a culinary perspective.

Chia seeds have received a lot of attention lately. These little black and white seeds were a major component of ancient Mayan and Aztec cultures. Chia seeds are reported to enhance and improve your energy level and physical stamina. While these claims have not been substantiated, their health benefits are undeniable. They contain twice as much protein as most other nuts or seeds as well as lots of calcium, omega-3 fatty acids, and anti-oxidants. They also contain lots of soluble fiber which causes them to swell rapidly. When this occurs in your stomach, it can induce satiety as well as slow down your intestine's absorption of sugar. Chia seeds are also reasonably priced compared to many other specialty health foods.

Nuts are Nature's Snack Food

Several studies have demonstrated the seemingly paradoxical effect of weight loss caused by eating high calorie nuts. Although nuts are very high in calories - even higher than what is found in most refined carbohydrate snacks - they typically do not result in weight gain. These results have been repeated in dozens of studies examining people's diets across world. It is clear that nuts have a thermostat lowering effect that prevents them from contributing to weight gain despite their high number of calories.

As you continue to enhance and further improve your diet, you'll begin to recognize that some foods have a powerful ability to control your appetite and reduce your cravings for processed snack foods. Without question, nuts are one of the most powerful plant based appetite suppressants. The need to snack is unavoidable. The decision over a lifetime is not whether or not you should snack on nuts – it's when you do snack, what makes the best choice? Since it is inevitable that you will continue to snack between meals, it is best to have a clear plan for the safest foods to eat when you do.

One or two ounces of nuts daily will enhance your weight loss, improve the overall health of your diet, and allow you to snack safely. Some people can eat large amounts of nuts daily without gaining weight, while others cannot. Since nuts won't raise your thermostat, the excess calories merely shift you from the starved side to the overfed side of your set point. The extra pounds caused by excessive nut intake will be much easier to shed than those brought on by high calorie, thermostat raising processed foods. If you are eating a lot of nuts and aren't meeting your weight loss goals, this should be one of the first places to cut back.

As you move further along through the program, nuts will help you maintain the changes that you've made so far. They offer a safe indulgence that you can implement into your diet every day that will not interfere with your weight loss efforts. Make sure that you are eating raw or natural nuts: not roasted, salted, blanched, or sweetened ones. During this station, experiment with nut based salad dressings and try to come up with your own versions. Integrating nuts into your diet will help you to achieve the goal of the next station - to limit junk food.

Summary

- The preparation of nuts determines how healthy they are - not the type of nut.
- Explore the nut-based salad dressings in the recipe section.
- Nuts make an ideal snack food.
- Nuts lower most people's set point.

Station 6 – Limit the Junk

Limit your intake of processed food to 1-2 servings per week.

Processed (or junk) food is everywhere. Processed
food is also very addictive. If you are overweight, it's very
likely that your body is particularly susceptible to the
thermostat raising effects of processed food, compared to
your thinner friends. We've already addressed the sugar, so
now it's time to attack the chips, pretzels, dips, fried foods,
salad dressings, white breads, yogurts, pastas and breakfast
cereals that work to keep your thermostat's set point high.

What is Junk Food?

Before we discuss strategies to limit processed (a.k.a.
junk) food, it's important that we define it. Processed food is
described as any food that is made from heavily manipulated
or altered natural ingredients. Processed food is usually high
in calories, carbohydrates, fat or sugar but does not have any
nutritional value. This makes them very calorie dense foods
opposed to the nutrient dense foods we are striving to eat
more of. Common processed foods include salted snack
foods like potato and corn chips, fried foods, and carbonated
beverages. All sweetened foods can be considered
processed, but we've already addressed them in Station 3.
Although most people don't think of white bread products

and pastas as processed foods, they should be considered as such since they contain lots of calories and very little nutrition.

Processed food comes from refining corn, soybeans, wheat, rice and potatoes into easily digestible chemicals that taste great and have a long shelf life. Processed food is fairly easy to spot if you look closely at the ingredient list. Here are some warning signs that a food is heavily processed and should be avoided.

- Sugar (also listed as maltose, dextrose, cane juice, high fructose corn syrup, fructose, sucrose or glucose) is one of the first four ingredients.
- The food contains more than 7 ingredients.
- Its "Sell By" Date is more than one month away.
- The list of ingredients contains lots of words that you can't pronounce.
- The list of ingredients contains any of the following: enriched flour, high fructose corn syrup, hydrogenated oils, corn oil, soybean oil, soy lecithin, nitrates, or xantham gum.
- The food is intended to be eaten as a snack, not part of a meal

On your next trip to the grocery store, apply this new, expanded definition to your usual staples. You'll find that most breakfast cereals, frozen dinners, breads, and side dishes are processed. Once you recognize how encompassing this new definition is, you'll soon realize that most of what Americans consume is processed food – on average 5 servings per day. It's likely that you'll discover that many foods that you always considered reasonable choices (breakfast cereals, granola bars, salad dressings, peanut butter, and frozen dinners) are in reality, junk food. Accepting that most of the food that the average American eats on a daily basis is junk is one of the most important steps to understanding what must be done to lose the weight and keep it off.

Once you eliminate these foods from your diet, you'll find that your grocery store trips take much less time. It is no longer necessary to go up and down every aisle since most of the aisles contain nothing but processed food. However, since you are buying more fruits and vegetables to replace the processed food, you'll have to increase the frequency of your trips. Your diet is now more perishable and it's impossible to buy fruits and vegetables that last for the whole week. If more frequent trips to the grocery store are not possible, look for frozen and canned versions of fruits and vegetables (read the labels carefully first) that offer a more convenient alternative to relying solely on fresh produce.

Junk Food: How Much is Too Much?

A complete avoidance of processed food is certainly a wonderful goal, though it is not realistic for most people. One of the distinct advantages of the *Pound of Cure* eating plan compared to most conventional diets is that it does not require 100% compliance to be effective. Because of the thermostat lowering power of this high nutrient diet, if you do stray from your eating plan a few times a week, you will still lose weight and improve your health. On a high nutrient diet like the *Pound of Cure* plan, excess calories are less likely to be stored as fat. This differs significantly from most low calorie or low carbohydrate diets where the slightest infraction stops your weight loss dead in its tracks. Your metabolism will not slow down because your weight loss is the result of a downward shift of your set point, not a migration away from it. In fact, if the food is having its desired effect and nudging your set point downward, your natural tendencies to burn off excess calories through an increased metabolism will be maintained as the pounds melt away.

It's impossible to make a blanket statement about a tolerable amount of processed food that will still allow weight loss since everyone responds differently to these foods and all processed foods are not created equally. A general starting point is to limit your processed food intake to 1-2 servings per week. If you exercise vigorously, are young, or are consuming much more than one pound of vegetables daily you may be able to tolerate more. Others may find that even at 1-2 servings per week, they are still unable to lose weight. Regardless of what your tolerance for processed food is, one thing is clear – the less of it you eat, the more weight you will lose.

Processed Food is Addictive

Processed food is highly addictive and can trigger a spike in your blood sugar that can result in a repetitive cycle that drives you to eat more. To demonstrate this, let's examine your blood sugar and insulin levels after you eat a junk food meal for breakfast. Let's consider pancakes and syrup as an example (which you'll quickly realize is a bad choice for breakfast). The figure below helps to illustrate the changes in your body's blood sugar over time after eating junk food.

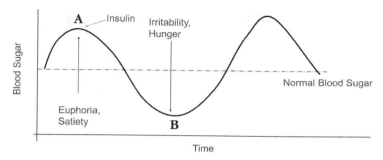

Figure 3 - Blood sugar after eating processed food

Immediately after you eat the pancakes, your blood sugar level begins to rise to Point A. This rise occurs very quickly since the pancakes are made of processed wheat flour that contains very little fiber, allowing your intestines to absorb it rapidly. At point A, you will start to feel happy since the high blood sugar triggers the pleasure centers in your brain. You will feel full and satisfied. However, as your blood sugar rises, it also triggers your pancreas to release insulin; rapid rises in blood sugar trigger lots of insulin to be released.

Insulin's primary goal is to keep the blood sugar at an even level. High blood sugars are not good for your body. Insulin tells your cells to pull the sugar out of the blood and ship it off to the liver and fat cells where it will be converted to fat and stored. This results in a rapid drop in your blood sugar level as all the carbohydrate that you've eaten leaves your blood stream to be stored as body fat. When the initial blood sugar spike is high and comes on quickly, the insulin tends to cause your blood sugar to overshoot the normal level, making it reach a lower than normal value, lower than before you ate. This brings us to point "B." You're now irritable because having a low blood sugar is no fun at all and of course, low blood sugar triggers your hunger drive just 60-90 minutes after you finished your meal. Suddenly that donut in the break room looks much more appealing.

Many people repeat this cycle 6-8 times in a single day, feeling as if they're unable to control their cravings. And, with each cycle, they are storing the ingested carbohydrate as body fat. Your craving for a midnight snack may be caused by a cycle that started that morning at the breakfast table. This repetitive cycle of blood sugar surges that trigger your brain's pleasure centers followed by a crash in the blood sugar and the accompanying cravings for more processed food demonstrates the addictive nature of processed food.

Junk Food Affects Us Differently

There is ample research that demonstrates that people's biologic response to processed food is different. Some people may not generate high insulin levels and rapid fat storage after eating processed food, while others may develop it after eating even healthy, nutrient dense foods.

Diabetes has reached epidemic levels in this country, affecting 11% of all adults and 27% of all senior citizens. The coincidence of diabetes and obesity has caused many in the medical community to refer to the syndrome of excess body weight and increased blood sugar as "diabesity." As diabesity worsens, patients go from needing only dietary changes to control blood sugar levels to requiring medications in pill form and ultimately needing insulin injections.

The point at which a diabetic is first placed on insulin injections can be a crucial moment in the course of the disease. Insulin is a very powerful thermostat raising hormone. This is not surprising since its primary function in the human body is to cause carbohydrates to be stored as fat. We see the thermostat raising effects whenever diabetic patients are first placed on insulin injections. The insulin usually results in significant, unpreventable weight gain which serves to worsen the disease that is being treated.

There are only two reasonable options for individuals who are overweight and require insulin to control their diabetes. The first is to follow a program like The *Pound of Cure* and change their eating habits to favor fruits and vegetables over processed foods. The other is to find a good bariatric surgeon and undergo a gastric bypass operation which will likely result in the immediate control of your blood sugars and prevent the need for starting insulin injections.

Now that we understand that processed foods stimulate the release of insulin and diabetics gain weight after starting insulin injections, a mechanism of the thermostat raising effects of processed foods becomes clear. These foods are uniquely able to stimulate insulin release which raises your thermostat's set point. The increased set point increases your true hunger signals and is coupled with the blood sugar swings that drive food cravings.

Station 6 is about stopping the cycle of rising and falling blood sugar levels throughout the day and putting an end to the unnecessary fat storage caused by thermostat raising processed foods. Although you may crave it for a few days or even weeks after you cut it out of your life, you'll be amazed at how little you miss it. Be sure to replace your processed food snacks with healthy fruits, nuts, and vegetables.

Summary

- Processed (a.k.a. junk) foods have calories but no nutrition – they are very calorie dense.
- People respond to junk food differently. Some are more susceptible to the thermostat raising impact of processed foods than others.
- Junk foods cause fluctuations in your insulin and blood sugar levels which can result in toxic food cravings.
- Junk foods also work to increase your true hunger and slow your metabolism by raising your thermostat's set point.

Station 7 – Starchy Vegetables and Grains

Limit wheat, corn starch, and white rice in your diet to once or twice per month. Limit yourself to one serving of colorless starchy vegetables daily, or one serving of whole grains daily.

For years, the American Heart Association (AHA) has urged us to eat more healthy whole grains. The bottom of the 1992 USDA food pyramid recommends 6-11 servings of bread, cereal, rice, and pasta. The origin of this advice is unclear and there is abundant evidence of the dangers of a diet high in grains. It's likely that this advice was based more on politics than on nutrition (grain farming is big business). The USDA has discontinued the entire concept of a food pyramid and now does not make any specific recommendations about grains except to recommend that at least half of the grains that you eat are whole grains.

The debate over the effectiveness of a low carbohydrate diet continues forty years after Dr. Atkins published his first book. Low carbohydrate diets have recently received some vindication after decades of derision by the medical community. Nonetheless, most people's experience with the diet that encourages steak, bacon, and cheese and scorns fruits and vegetables has been mixed at best. Exceptionally few people have found that a high fat, low carb lifestyle resulted in long term, durable weight loss.

Although the *Pound of Cure* program does not encourage the intake of grains, even unprocessed whole grains, it is not a low carbohydrate diet. The truth, as many of us have come to realize, is that some carbohydrates are good for weight loss and others are not. It should come as no surprise that fruits, grains, processed foods, and sugars all have different effects on your metabolic thermostat.

Carbohydrates can come in many forms. We've already discussed the processed foods that make up the majority of America's carbohydrate intake. Obviously these foods should be limited as much as possible. Fruits are another source of carbohydrates (fructose), which we've demonstrated makes an excellent food choice. Beans will be discussed later, but their presence on The Metabolic Reset Program shows us that they are an important part of your diet.

This station will focus on both starchy vegetables (potatoes, beets, squash, etc.) and whole grains. It also addresses the particular dangers of wheat, white rice, and corn starch. Although some starchy vegetables and a little whole grains in your diet are acceptable, eating large quantities will sabotage your weight loss goals. If you are not trying to lose weight, and only want to eat healthier, starchy vegetables can be eaten in unlimited quantities. Whole grains should still be limited to one or two servings daily.

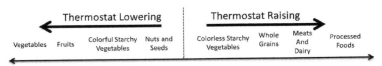

Figure 4 - Thermostat Raising and Lowering Foods

In truth, the thermostat effects of starchy vegetables and grains differ significantly. Colorful starchy vegetables are typically high in nutrition and fiber and fall toward the end of the nutrient density spectrum. They make good food choices and can usually be eaten in unlimited amounts. Colorless starchy vegetables do not have more calories than their colorful cousins. However, they typically contain less nutrition, making them more calorie dense, and therefore, a less optimal food choice. It's impossible to make a blanket statement about how an entire class of foods impacts your thermostat since this will vary from person to person.

Whole grains like oats (either steel cut or rolled), brown rice, quinoa and millet have received a tremendous amount of attention in the media and are touted as being good for your heart and your waistline. Despite this positive attention, the evidence does not support the claims. Wheat, the most commercial of all foods and a staple of the western diet, has a dangerous impact on our health and well-being and should be avoided as much as possible.

Colorful, starchy vegetables *(unlimited)*	Whole grains and colorless starchy vegetables *(once daily)*	Processed Grains *(1-2x per month)*
		Corn Starch
Beets	Barley	**Wheat**
Pumpkin	Buckwheat	White Rice
Sweet Potatoes	Brown Rice	
Squash, Acorn	Corn	
Squash, Butternut	Jicama	
Yams	Millet	
	Oats	
	Parsnips	
	Popcorn	
	Quinoa	
	Rye	
	Spelt	
	Turnips	
	White Potatoes	

Most people will do well eating one serving of colorless starchy vegetables or whole grains daily. Processed grains should be avoided. The vibrant colors of beets, pumpkins, sweet potatoes, squash, and yams are a giveaway that they are packed with nutrition. The high nutritional value of these foods makes them the most thermostat lowering of all the foods listed. Although they may contain a similar amount of calories to the other foods, the greater nutritional value makes them more satisfying and better choices overall.

Whole Grains and the Glycemic Index

Despite all the health benefits of "healthy whole grains" that the USDA and AHA report, there is little evidence to support these claims and a good deal of evidence that demonstrates the harmful effects of these foods. While you don't have to completely avoid whole grains, it is important to recognize their harmful effects on your metabolic thermostat and their ability to slow your weight loss if eaten in large amounts.

The popularity of the South Beach Diet and other programs that rely on a principle known as the glycemic index has given Americans the impression that whole grains make great food choices. Many of the large food producers have latched on to the whole grains concept and use it as an effective marketing tool. There are even advertisements that tout several well-known sugar cereals as being high in whole grains.

The glycemic index principle states that some carbohydrates cause your blood glucose to rise rapidly while others cause less of a rise. It is only applicable to carbohydrates, not proteins or fats. Theoretically, those carbohydrate foods that cause only a small rise in your blood sugar are less fattening than those that cause a rapid rise. This principle supports eating whole wheat bread and steel-cut oatmeal liberally while avoiding white bread and instant oatmeal since the latter group causes a higher spike in your blood sugar and, therefore, has a higher glycemic index.

Although the glycemic index does have some value in determining the thermostat effects of different carbohydrates, we have to be careful with the assumptions that we make. Those unprocessed whole grains that have a lower glycemic index will trigger less insulin release than high glycemic index grains will. In the previous station, we identified insulin as a very powerful thermostat raising hormone. It follows that since whole grains cause less insulin release, they cause less of a rise in your thermostat's set point. Advocates of whole grains interpret this statement as "not causing **any** increase," as opposed to the more accurate interpretation of causing **less** of an increase in your set point.

Because our metabolic thermostat is controlled by many more factors than just insulin levels, a strict reliance on the glycemic index underestimates the impact of grains on our waistline and unfairly vilifies some fruits that are loaded with nutrition like melons, mangoes, and pineapples. In my practice, I don't rely heavily on glycemic index values to determine whether foods make good weight loss choices.

The current whole grains fad is primarily being driven through the marketing efforts of the large food producers. Grain production offers manufacturers the opportunity to convert a nickel's worth of raw grains into a box of cereal that can be sold for $4.99. The profitability of these foods brings into question the validity of the marketing campaigns that extol the virtues of whole grains. The only way that eating whole grains can be proven to be a good food choice is when it is compared to processed grains. It's never mentioned that, compared to beans, legumes, vegetables, and fruits, whole grains make poor food choices. Only because most American's eat processed grains in large amounts is there any benefit to adopting a whole grain based diet. In my office, I compare whole grain foods to low tar cigarettes – even though low tar cigarettes make better choices than their full tar versions, it doesn't mean that you should smoke them.

Wheat

Although the presence of corn starch and white rice on a list of foods to avoid would not surprise most people, the inclusion of wheat is often received with an audible gasp. There is, perhaps, no food considered more American than wheat. "Amber waves of grain" are sung about in America the Beautiful - perhaps one of the most loved patriotic songs second only to our National Anthem. Wheat is grown on more land area than any other commercial crop and is considered one of the most important foods in our diet. It is written about in the bible and plays an important role in the ceremonies of most of the currently practiced religions. Whole wheat breads have been marketed as the choice that "health nuts" make and are perceived as good food choices.

Today's wheat is much different than wheat produced fifty years ago. Today's wheat is a result of genetic hybridization. Wheat plants have been cultivated and bred to provide a greater yield over the last few decades. The reality is that today's wheat plants cannot survive in the wild unassisted - it can only grow if it is provided with nitrates for fertilizer and other human interventions.

Wheat is more heavily traded than all other crops combined and this commercialization has driven extensive genetic manipulation in order to improve our ability to grow it efficiently. Today's genetically modified wheat contains properties that make it particularly dangerous to your health.

Gluten, the main protein in wheat, is broken down by your intestines into a compound called gliadin that has a powerful impact on your thermostat's set point. Also, the byproducts of wheat ingestion include extremely addictive compounds called exorphins that trigger the same centers of your brain as opiate drugs like morphine and heroin.

There have been several studies that demonstrate that people who eat wheat gliadin will ingest, on average, 400 calories per day more than those who don't take in any of this compound. The digestion of other grains does not produce the exorphins that are released when we ingest hybridized wheat.

Wheat's effect on your brain can be demonstrated by using the drug Naloxone which blocks the pleasure centers of the brain. In several experiments, subjects who were given Naloxone prior to a wheat based meal ate 30% fewer calories than those who did not receive the drug. When people stop eating wheat, there is usually a 3-4 day period of withdrawal characterized by headaches, short attention span, and depression. You may have experienced these symptoms when you were on the Metabolic Reset Program.

Although sprouted wheat bread (a.k.a. Ezekiel bread) is a better alternative to whole wheat, it still contains loads of gluten and has the same addictive and appetite stimulant effects. Many gluten free products also contain corn starch, tapioca starch, and potato starch that are only slightly less harmful to your metabolism than wheat flour. These products should be avoided.

Wheat works through two synergistic mechanisms to cause weight gain. First, the gliadin acts to raise your thermostat, thus increasing your true hunger. Second, the gluten is metabolized into exorphins that trigger the pleasure sensors in your brain which results in toxic food cravings.

This same two-pronged attack on our hunger is seen with junk foods and represents a unique threat to our ability to make good food choices and lose weight.

Eliminating wheat from your diet is a far more demanding change than limiting starchy vegetables and other grains. I urge you to make a two week commitment to a wheat free diet. If you begin to experience headaches and other withdrawal symptoms, resist the temptation to relieve them by eating wheat. These symptoms are not a sign of your body's need for wheat and are only temporary. Those people with the most severe withdrawal symptoms usually obtain the most significant benefit from a wheat free diet. After you complete your two weeks of wheat free living, you'll likely notice that your food cravings have decreased and it's very likely that you've lost a few pounds as well.

Cutting down on your starchy vegetables and grains and eliminating wheat will further your need to eat lots of vegetables, fruit, beans, legumes, nuts, seeds, and lean animal proteins to satisfy your appetite. Focus on these foods and within a few weeks, your desire for wheat will be a distant memory.

Summary

- Colorful, starchy vegetables can usually be eaten in unlimited quantities.
- Whole grains raise your thermostat's set point and should be limited. They do not represent good food choices.
- Wheat should be avoided as much as possible due to its powerful set point raising effects and ability to induce toxic food cravings.
- The glycemic index is not a useful measure of how fattening a food is.

Station 8 – Limit Dairy

Limit your intake of dairy to 2-3 servings per week or fewer. Limit cheese consumption to 1-2 servings per month. Any dairy products consumed should be labeled "No rBGH."

Whether or not dairy is a useful addition to our diet is a very hotly debated point among nutritionists. In order to understand whether dairy is a good food choice, it's important to understand the business behind the dairy industry.

The dairy industry is made up of a small handful of multi-billion dollar corporations, and many are located outside of the U.S. These few corporations are responsible for producing more than half the milk consumed in the United States. These very powerful groups of dairy farmers have put a great deal of money and effort into convincing Americans that dairy products are a critical part of a healthy diet, and without cow's milk we are likely to become obese, calcium deficient, and develop osteoporosis.

A class action lawsuit was filed in 2005 by the Physicians Committee for Responsible Medicine that attacked the dairy industry's claim that consuming dairy results in weight loss. The claim that eating dairy is an effective way to lose weight was based on two, very small scale, poorly conducted studies that were funded by the Dairy Council.

The result of the class action lawsuit was that the dairy industry was forced to halt their advertising campaign that claimed that eating a diet rich in dairy resulted in weight loss. However, the effects of this advertising campaign persist and most of the world looks at dairy as an important part of a healthy diet. Unfortunately, it is not; and the less dairy you eat, the more likely you are to lose the weight.

Americans Eat Too Much Dairy

When working with overweight patients who are having difficulty losing weight despite eating what they perceive is a healthy diet, the cause of the poor weight loss is frequently too much dairy. Because we've been convinced that low fat cheese, yogurt, and low calorie ice cream desserts make good choices, we've overeaten these foods without realizing their effect on our thermostat. The reason that overeating dairy products causes weight gain is clear when you look at what they are made of: lactose (a sugar) and milk fat. Dairy products, like yogurt, obtain most of their calories from the sugar component, while the calories in cheese come predominantly from the fat component. Milk and cottage cheese are a more even mix of sugar and fat calories.

Lactose has a low glycemic index, meaning that it does not result in a rapid increase in your blood sugar after you eat it. What we've discovered in the last station remains true: the glycemic index can be misleading. This statement is particularly true when the glycemic index is used to determine the impact of sugars on our waist-line.

The glycemic index only considers the impact of food on blood sugar levels and does not account for the level of sugar in your liver. Lactose, like most sugars, is heavily metabolized in the liver and does not result in a spike in your blood sugar since the carbohydrate is immediately converted to fat in the liver.

Remember that the only food that contains sugar and does not raise your thermostat is fruit. The reason that fruit does not raise your set point is because it is also packaged with fiber and loads of micronutrients. The sugar in milk is not packaged with fiber and contains none of the magical, undiscovered antioxidants and other nutrients that we find in fruits and vegetables. Because the poisonous sugar in milk is not packaged with an antidote (fiber), your metabolic thermostat is allowed to inch upward by a very small amount with every serving.

The calories in many dairy products come primarily from fat rather than protein as you might assume from the way it is labeled. Most cheese gets as much as 90% of its calories from fat, implying that eating cheese is not that much different than eating plain butter. Even the reduced fat varieties of cheese obtain 60% of their calories from fat. Because of the very addictive, rich taste of cheese and the high calorie density, you should minimize your intake of cheese to only a few servings per month. Even reduced fat versions should be viewed with skepticism and not looked at as healthy food choices.

Protein Shakes

Whey protein shakes have been popular weight loss tools for over thirty years. Recently, the variety and consumption of whey protein shakes has increased significantly. It is now possible to purchase whey protein shakes in nearly every grocery, convenience and drug store in the United States. Whey protein shakes were popularized by the Slimfast® diet which promoted a shake for breakfast and lunch instead of eating real food. The recent use of whey protein shakes to obtain rapid weight loss for pre-operative bariatric surgery patients and as a transition back to regular food in postoperative patients has likely fueled their resurgence in popularity. Although the shakes are useful in the bariatric surgery population, their utility in non-surgical patients is minimal.

Even as a bariatric surgeon who relies heavily on whey protein shakes in the immediate postoperative phase, I try to wean my patients from them as quickly as possible and do not encourage their use for the long term. When treating patients for weight loss who aren't considering surgery, I never use them.

A diet in which breakfast and lunch are replaced by a protein shake typically results in a low calorie diet – usually between 800-1000 calories per day. As we've come to realize, starvation diets will never result in durable weight loss. When patients resume their previous eating habits, the weight is almost immediately regained. Also, protein shakes are artificially flavored and sweetened and contain a long list of unpronounceable ingredients. Many of these ingredients have thermostat raising properties, which shift your set point upward. The result is an even greater magnification of the typical starvation metabolic responses. As your weight drops from the calorie restriction and your set point shifts upward, you will experience even greater hunger and a slower metabolism than usual. The result is inevitable. Ultimately you'll break down and find yourself in the midst of a massive eating binge and when the weight comes back on, you'll have a few extra pounds as a result of your higher set point.

Protein bars are even more dangerous to your weight loss success. Frequently, these bars are little more than candy bars with whey protein powder added. If it seems too good to be true, it probably is. Eating a bar made of chocolate and caramel will not help you lose weight in the long run. You should completely eliminate the protein bars and shakes from your weight loss plan. They are processed, artificially (and sometimes sugar-) sweetened foods that will not help you on your search for durable weight loss.

Calcium

The primary nutritional claim that keeps us shopping in the dairy aisle at the supermarket is its ability to provide calcium for healthy bones. Despite the fact that the United States consumes more dairy than almost any other country, our rate of osteoporosis continues to climb. If you live to the age of 85, you have a 30% chance of suffering a hip fracture at some point in your life. Hip fractures are usually caused by falls which are more related to your functional status (discussed in Station 4) than to bone density.

Contrary to popular belief, you can maintain good bone health without eating dairy. All fruits and vegetables contain calcium, and your current diet of over a pound of vegetables daily and at least four servings of fruit daily will provide you with all the calcium your bones need. Kale, bok-choy, collard greens, sesame seeds, turnip greens, and spinach all contain particularly high amounts of calcium. Many have more calcium per serving than milk does. There are two other reasons that obtaining your calcium from vegetables is better than getting it from dairy products. First, the calcium in vegetables is more readily absorbable. Your intestinal tract is better able to transport the calcium from vegetables into your bloodstream and ultimately into your bones than it is for the calcium found in dairy. Second, a diet rich in animal fat and animal protein (i.e. dairy) creates an acid load on your kidneys. Your kidneys will use calcium as a means to buffer this acid load and as a result you will excrete more calcium in your urine than you will if your diet does not contain large amounts of animal fat and protein. The end result is that your *Pound of Cure* diet actually lowers your calcium requirements since you'll be excreting less calcium in your urine. Eating a diet rich in dairy and therefore animal fat increases your calcium needs. This hamster wheel effect in which eating more calcium in the form of dairy increases your need for more calcium explains the increasing rate of osteoporosis despite America's mass consumption of dairy products.

Hormones in Dairy Products

The safety of dairy products has been continually brought into question due to the practice of administering hormones to cows in order to increase their milk production. The primary hormone in question is a drug called rBGH - a growth hormone that stimulates cows' udders to grow and produce additional milk. Many critics of the use of rBGH claim that it increases the rate of infection in cows' udders (mastitis) which can result in contamination of the milk by bacteria. It also results in higher levels of a compound called IGF-1 in the milk. IGF-1 has been labeled as a carcinogen in many countries. The mountain of evidence that supports this claim grows as rapidly as the dairy industry funded research that refutes it. The battles in court between several consumer safety organizations and the makers of the hormone continues to escalate. Most European nations and Canada have banned the use of rBGH due to the suspicion that the milk that comes from cows treated with this hormone causes cancer. When you do indulge in dairy products, make sure to look for those labeled "No rBGH."

Dairy Alternatives

Before you give up on milk in your morning coffee, there are some dairy alternatives that are high in calcium, low in calories, and just as delicious as cow's milk. Most supermarkets now offer rice milk, soy milk, coconut milk, and almond milk as alternatives to dairy products. Rice milk tends to be high in carbohydrates and coconut milk is high in fat. Of the two, coconut milk is a better choice and is a commonly used ingredient in some of the nut based salad dressings mentioned previously.

Soy and almond milks make good choices. Soy milk contains almost as much calcium as cow's milk and approximately the same number of calories as skim milk. However, too much soy can inhibit your thyroid function and mimic high estrogen levels which can raise your thermostat's setting. Nonetheless, if you limit your soy intake to once per day, you should not experience these harmful effects. The clear winner in the milk alternative race is almond milk - it's high in calcium, low in calories, and tastes delicious. It's available at most grocery stores and should help you to keep your intake of dairy to a minimum.

When choosing a brand of almond milk, look for unsweetened versions and read the labels carefully since some brands contain added sugars and artificial sweeteners. Finally, be wary of non-dairy creamers since most are very high in sugar, high fructose corn syrup, and are not acceptable dairy alternatives.

Many patients who are struggling to lose weight can get the scale moving in the right direction by cutting back on dairy. Dairy products contain lactose which is more fattening than its glycemic index would lead you to believe and are typically much higher in fat than we appreciate. The reasoning behind America's belief that dairy products are necessary for good health - calcium - is overstated. Good bone health can be easily achieved by eating a diet rich in fruits and vegetables. Finally, today's milk comes from hormone-treated cows and is not nearly as healthy as we'd like to believe. Cut back on your dairy intake to 2-3 servings per week and keep your cheese intake to 1-2 servings per month and you'll continue to shed the pounds and improve your health.

Summary

- Dairy consists primarily of fat and sugar.
- Protein shakes are not good food choices and should not play a role in your long term weight loss efforts.
- Dairy is not necessary for bone health. Fruits and vegetables are better sources for calcium.
- Almond milk, coconut milk, and soy milk are suitable alternatives to dairy with almond milk being the ideal choice.

Station 9 – Cut Down on Animal Protein

Limit your intake of animal protein to 4-8 ounces per day. Avoid industrial raised beef and eggs completely, favoring grass fed beef and eggs from a local farm. Limit fish intake to one serving per week except for shellfish and small, oily fish like anchovies, herring, and sardines. Eat lots of beans, lentils and legumes, but limit soy intake to one serving per day. Avoid synthetic protein shakes and bars.

For decades, the vegetarian community has lived on the fringe of the nutritional world with the majority of vegetarians having made the choice not to eat meat based on ethical and moral grounds rather than nutritional ones. In 2004, a book by T. Colin Campbell, *The China Study*, changed all of that. The book revealed the findings of the largest study on human nutrition that has ever been performed (and likely ever will be).

The China-Cornell-Oxford Project was a twenty-year study that examined the mortality rates from cancer, and other chronic diseases, of people from 65 counties in rural China. Rural China is a unique place to perform nutritional studies because there is wide variation in the diet of its citizens from county to county due to its natural resources. Also, people tend to live their entire lifetime in the same place they were born. A similar study could never be performed in the U.S. because we all eat very similarly (bad), and it is common for people to move throughout the country several times during their lifetime.

The investigators of the China-Cornell-Oxford Project conclude that a vegan diet - which avoids meats, fish, and dairy products - prevents most cancers and chronic diseases. They go so far as to declare animal protein a "carcinogen." They also claim that the majority of Western diseases could be completely eliminated if Americans would subscribe to a vegan diet.

To his credit, Dr. Campbell made the data he used to draw his conclusions available to the public. Re-analysis of this data has illustrated several issues in Dr. Campbell's statistics and has pointed to the intake of grains as a greater cause of Western ailments such as heart disease, diabetes, and obesity. The debate over whether grains or animal protein are the primary culprit in our society's deteriorating health rages on.

Supporters of the China study's conclusion that a vegan diet provides the greatest amount of protection from chronic disease include two popular nutritionists: Dean Ornish, MD and Jeff Fuhrman, MD. Dr. Ornish has advocated a lifestyle driven approach to the treatment of heart disease rather than the medication and procedure based approach that most physicians advocate. He claims that he can reverse heart disease through a vegan diet, moderate exercise, yoga, and meditation. He has published extensively about his program and it is widely accepted that there is merit to his treatment plan; however, it has not been widely adopted by most doctors.

Dr. Fuhrman has coined the formula: Health = Nutrients/Calories, advocating for a nutrient dense eating style (like the *Pound of Cure* approach). Although there are critics of Dr. Campbell, Ornish, and Fuhrman, it is difficult to argue that animal protein is healthy – even the strongest critics argue that it is "equivalent" to vegetable based proteins and "not harmful." The advice to avoid eating meat is met with strong resistance from many people who would never adopt a vegetarian diet regardless of the health benefits. Although cutting out animal protein entirely will result in an extremely healthy eating style, it is not necessary to achieve significant weight loss and health benefits. By changing the amount and - as important - the type of meat, fish, and poultry that you eat, you can achieve nearly the same results as those obtained from a strict vegan diet.

What did your meat eat?

Animal proteins have been stratified in the popular press in terms of their nutritional value, with fish being thought of as the healthiest option, chicken and other poultry as second healthiest and red meat options like beef and lamb the least healthy. Unfortunately, the actual nutritional value of these animal proteins is not nearly so clear cut. In order to determine the healthfulness of animal protein you must consider what the animal ate when it was alive. Cows (like humans) develop large stores of fat in their body when they are fed a diet of primarily grain. And, when Cows (like humans) eat a primarily green vegetable diet (grass), they develop lean muscle without much body fat. This fact explains the difference between pastured (a.k.a. grass fed) beef and traditional industrial beef.

Cows that are allowed to roam freely on a green pasture and eat grass result in beef that is leaner, lower in saturated fats and higher in healthy omega-3 fats than their industrial grain fed counterparts. Additionally, grass fed cows do not typically require antibiotics because their grass fed diet and lack of confinement make them much less susceptible to disease. Finally, grass fed cows are typically not given hormones and take more than twice as long to grow to a mature size before they are slaughtered (which explains the increased price).

Let's look closer at the hormones that are given to industrial raised cows to speed up their growth rate. It is now clear that these hormones must have the same impact on cows' thermostat set points that medications like corticosteroids and insulin have on ours. The growth hormones given to cows stimulate their hunger and decrease their metabolic rate. It is possible that we are ingesting small amounts of these hormones when we eat the beef that comes from industrial raised cows. It is very concerning that the residual levels of growth hormones present in industrial raised beef may affect our thermostats in the same way.

There are similar differences in chickens that are raised in an unconfined state – both the poultry meat and their eggs are far healthier than the less expensive industrial raised options. Although there are significant differences in the quality of the poultry meat, the greater difference lies in the quality of the eggs. Eggs that come from chickens allowed to roam freely and eat a natural diet (grubs and grass) are more flavorful and higher in healthy omega-3 fats than eggs from industrial raised chickens. Although there are several different labels that are meant to indicate that they were raised humanely (cage free, free range, and 100% organic), these eggs do not compare to those that come directly from a local farm. When shopping for eggs, look for words like "rotational grazing" or a stamp from a farm a short drive away. The yolks of these eggs will be a vibrant orange color rather than the typical yellow hue that you are used to.

Fish

While beef and poultry offer healthy alternatives to industrial farming techniques, fish remain a more difficult problem. Although fish contain a very favorable amount of healthy omega-3 fats, there are downsides to both farmed and wild fish. Farmed fish are typically raised in confinement off shorelines, or more recently in indoor facilities. The mercury content of these fish is lower (particularly in the indoor farmed varieties), making them better choices than their wild counterparts. Mercury levels are so high in wild caught fish that you should limit your intake to just 2-3 times per month. Unfortunately, farm raised fish suffer from many of the same issues that industrial raised beef and poultry do; the fish are fed lower quality foods that differ significantly from the fish's natural diet, resulting in less favorable nutritional profiles.

Farm raised fish are susceptible to disease due to their cramped quarters and are typically administered antibiotics in their feed. Because of the high levels of mercury in wild caught fish and the poor nutritional profile of farm raised fish, it is best to limit your intake of all fish to once per week. The exception to this rule is the small, oily, wild-caught fish like sardines, herring, and anchovies. They contain little mercury due to their low position on the food chain and high levels of omega-3 fats. These small, oily fish can be eaten 2-3 times per week safely. Also, shellfish such as shrimp, clams, crabs, and oysters contain low levels of mercury and can be eaten safely several times per week.

Plant Sources of Protein

Cutting down on animal protein does not mean cutting down on protein altogether. In fact, it is critical that you replace the animal protein that you are no longer eating with plant based proteins. The best source of protein from plants comes from beans, lentils and legumes. These foods can be eaten in unlimited amounts without causing weight gain.

Although many people point to beans' high carbohydrate load as a factor that can result in weight gain, this is likely not the case. The majority of the carbohydrate in beans is not absorbed; rather it travels through your small intestine into your colon where it serves as fuel for the bacteria that live there. As the bacteria metabolize the carbohydrate, gas is released. The upside is that the carbohydrate in beans is only partially absorbed and therefore does not cause weight gain. The downside is that all the gas created by the bacteria results in flatulence. Regular intake of beans may initially cause increased abdominal bloating, however after a few weeks, this effect diminishes.

Soy is another vegetable source of protein. However, eating it in large amounts can cause hormonal and thyroid issues and large doses of soy may increase your thermostat's set point. Because of this, you should limit your intake of soy to one serving daily.

By limiting your intake of animal protein to 1-2 servings daily, and eating large amounts of vegetable proteins, you will stimulate weight loss and reduce your exposure to many of the chronic diseases that a diet rich in animal protein and fat cause. Given the small amount of animal protein that you do take in, you'll be able to afford the higher costs of quality grass fed beef and farm fresh eggs, eliminating the toxic effects of their industrial counterparts.

Summary

- Animal protein is thought by many to be the cause of most chronic diseases.
- The living conditions and diet of the animals are the primary determinant of the healthfulness of meat, fish, or poultry.
- Look for grass fed beef and farm fresh eggs instead of their industrial farmed counterparts.
- Animals that are administered hormones gain weight quickly. If meat from these animals contains significant levels of these substances, it could have a similar impact on those of us who consume them.
- Wild fish are high in mercury and farm raised fish are often treated with hormones and antibiotics. Limit your intake of all fish to 2-3 times per month.

Station 10 – Exercise for the Right Reasons

If you are physically capable, start a structured exercise program. Weight training and high intensity interval training are the best for weight loss, while moderate cardiovascular exercise helps relieve stress.

For decades, physicians and skinny friends alike have offered the over simplified, demeaning, and (what we now know) flat out wrong advice: eat less and exercise more. If things were this simple, obesity would be a temporary annoyance and not a life threatening, crippling disease. As you've learned so far, how much you eat is not nearly as important as what you eat. Now, we'll discuss the very limited role that exercise plays in your long-term weight loss goals.

Patients frequently complain that they're unable to lose weight because of an orthopedic problem that limits their ability to exercise. This is simply not true as weight loss is almost entirely dependent on your food intake and not the amount of exercise you do. There are exceptions to this rule that we'll discuss later, but for the most part, exercise is neither necessary nor important for you to meet your weight loss goals. Nonetheless, there are some very good reasons that you should participate in a structured exercise program, and for many it may be a critical component of your success - but not for the reasons you think.

Moderate Exercise Isn't Enough

The American Heart Association (AHA) recommends 150 minutes per week of moderate exercise or 75 minutes per week of vigorous exercise. This recommendation is strictly targeted at maintaining your cardiovascular health but has been widely adopted as the right recommendations for weight loss as well. Moderate exercise results in around 200-400 calories burned per hour depending on your weight and age. Meeting the AHA's guidelines would result in 500-1000 calories burned per week. These calories burned can be wiped out with one large meal.

Now that we have a better understanding of our body's metabolic thermostat, we recognize that moderate exercise will generally increase your appetite by an amount equal to the amount of calories burned - resulting in no net change in your calorie balance. The goal of any exercise program should not be to burn off calories during the exercise session but rather to lower your thermostat's set point by building muscle.

Although moderate exercise will burn some calories, your metabolic rate will go right back to normal within an hour or two. This fact proves that moderate exercise has very little impact on your thermostat and does not result in even a short lived improvement. Because there is no change in your set point, the number of calories that you burn on the treadmill will never make up for the increase in your appetite. That's right! Spend 45 minutes on the treadmill and you'll burn around 300 calories. If you finish up your workout routine with a bagel and cream cheese, you'll be no better off (from a weight loss perspective) then if you slept in and skipped the bagel. It's for this reason that following the AHA's guidelines will not aid you in your weight loss efforts. If you're trying to lose weight through exercise, you're going to have to do more than moderate exercise. You're going to have to work to build muscle and 45 minutes on the treadmill is not going to do it.

There is a significant variability in your body's response to exercise. Most young people (under 30) can achieve significant weight loss from an aggressive exercise regimen. Most of us start to lose muscle as we age, starting in our twenties. Building up your muscle mass is an uphill battle. Young people still have the physical ability to add a significant amount of muscle which will work to lower your set point. This does not mean that exercise represents a lost cause for the rest of us. All of us should exercise no matter what age or level of functional status. But, if your goal is weight loss, you should focus on building muscle which will help lower our thermostat's set point.

In my practice, I often see patients who have gained a lot of weight in their early adult years after spending their high school years slim and trim. Invariably, I find that in high school, these patients were active on their athletic teams, spending several hours a day performing vigorous exercise. They ate whatever they wanted and stayed thin because they were maintaining their thermostat's set point through exercise. After they graduated, their exercise level decreased precipitously resulting in a loss of muscle. The weight gain in these situations is rapid. The set point goes up and the appetite follows to increase the weight to this new, higher set point.

Young people who engage in an intense exercise program in order to lose or control their weight without making the necessary changes to their eating habits are very prone to weight regain. Any life event that results in an interruption of their exercise routine: an injury, job change, or birth of a child will likely result in very rapid weight gain. Even if you are able to lose a substantial amount of weight from exercise, it is very difficult to maintain it unless you make changes to your diet as well.

High Intensity Interval Training

A new exercise trend represents an improvement over the marginal weight loss results that moderate exercise provides. High Intensity Interval Training is a technique of 6-10 repetitions of 1-2 minute "sprints," forcing your heart rate up to 90% of its maximum. Each sprint is followed by a similar length period of moderate exercise for "rest." Although these exercise sessions typically last less than 30 minutes, they have demonstrated much higher levels of fat burning and performance enhancement than typical moderate exercise sessions. Even more impressive, several studies have demonstrated that your metabolic rate remains increased for up to 24 hours after a high intensity session compared to the almost immediate return to normal that we see after moderate exercise sessions. The prolonged elevation of your metabolic rate shows that interval training can lower your set point – at a least for a day or so.

Despite the benefits of high intensity training, it is not a technique that is right for everyone. First, before engaging in such a regimen, it is critical that you obtain clearance from your physician. It is probably best to have a stress test performed if you are over the age of forty or have any cardiovascular risk factors like high cholesterol, high blood pressure, or diabetes. Second, many patients are unable to participate in this level of exercise due to deconditioning or orthopedic limitations. Although it is possible to gradually integrate high intensity exercise into your routine, it should only be done with guidance from your physician and a skilled trainer.

When counseling patients, I never start with exercise. It represents only a small part of the solution and most are not able to participate in the type of program that is necessary given their current weight. It is only after a significant amount of weight loss that I begin to get people started on an exercise program. It's at this point that activities like high intensity interval training are possible.

The improved results offered by high intensity interval training have shed some light on the types of exercise that should be performed in order to lose weight. For decades, all recommendations have centered around moderate intensity exercise with the active discussions centered on the length of time necessary for optimal results. Our recent understanding of the more impressive benefits of vigorous exercise has changed this discussion significantly. It's likely that the most important determinant of the benefits of an exercise is the intensity rather than the duration. The popularity of programs like P90X® and CrossFit® are well deserved since they demand shorter bursts of more intense movements. If you are able to participate in a program that forces you to push yourself well beyond your normal levels of activity, you will achieve a greater increase in your strength and endurance - and most importantly - your thermostat's set point.

The next time you are watching a reality TV show about weight loss (i.e. Biggest Loser), watch what types of exercises are performed. The contestants aren't walking on the treadmill for hours on end. They're sprinting on the treadmill then immediately doing pushups, followed by climbing several flights of stairs and finally taking a break to dry heave in the corner from sheer exhaustion before hopping right back on the treadmill again. The exercise routines used in these shows represent the extreme end of the spectrum and are not recommended. However, they demonstrate that it is the intensity that matters when it comes to losing weight - not the duration.

Resistance Training (Weight Lifting)

Although the American Heart Association has not made significant changes in its exercise recommendations to accommodate our better understanding of the importance of building muscle, the American Diabetes Association (ADA) has. The ADA now recommends resistance training (weight lifting) at least two - but ideally - three times weekly along with regular aerobic exercise. These recommendations come from the improved insulin and blood sugar levels seen in patients after weight lifting. This comes as no surprise because of our understanding that building healthy muscle will lower your set point.

One of the most important parts of any weight lifting routine is to ensure that you use the proper technique when you exercise. All of us have seen young men writhing and squirming their way through a weight lifting exercise just so they can be seen lifting the heavier weights. This is foolish and leads to injury. It also offers little benefit. It is much better to choose lighter weights and employ perfect technique – you'll improve faster and will minimize your chance of injury. When getting started, a few sessions with a trainer can be invaluable. Make sure the trainer pays close attention to your form and offers constructive criticism to ensure that you are performing each movement precisely.

Exercise for Stress Relief

High intensity interval training and weight lifting will lower your thermostat's set point while moderate aerobic exercise probably will not. However, there is still one very important benefit to be obtained from any exercise regimen: stress release.

Stress is a very potent thermostat raising agent and if not appropriately dealt with, can result in permanent weight gain. It is likely that the impact of stress on our appetite, or what most of us refer to as "emotional eating," is actually the increased appetite that stress causes by raising our set point. Although I fully admit that our thermostat model cannot explain all eating behaviors, it is likely that there is more biology governing our tendency to eat when under stress than we've previously believed. Stress eating tends to worsen stress, not relieve it. If you are feeling stressed and indulge in a sugary, fattening dessert, you've accomplished nothing. The stressor remains unchanged and you've added the guilt and shame that goes along with your unhealthy indulgence. Plus, in 30-60 minutes, you'll experience a low blood sugar attack that causes your brain to magnify things even further.

Exercise, however, has the opposite effect. Exercise of any type releases endorphins that are very effective for minimizing stress. No problem seems as bad after an exercise session as it did before it. Those patients who feel daily stress (let's be honest, this is most of us) should begin an exercise routine for the sole purpose of managing their stress.

Finally, your exercise routine, whether it is moderate aerobics, high intensity intervals, or weight training should be fun. If you dread your daily workout, it's time to find a new routine. Exercise should make up the best part of your day - not the worst. Also, don't forget about basketball, soccer, tennis, volleyball, dance, indoor rock climbing, and other sports and activities that not only provide a great workout, but can also be a lot of fun.

Now that you have a better understanding of the true effects of exercise on your body, you can better select an appropriate routine for the right reason. If you are young and enjoy exercising, dive into a high intensity interval training program and push yourself to the limit. Just make sure that you honor the changes in your eating habits that you've made in the earlier stations and don't rely on exercise alone to meet your weight loss goals. If high intensity intervals seem like more than you can handle for now, start with a mixture of weight lifting and aerobic exercise. Begin using low weights, but don't be afraid to push yourself when you feel your strength improving. Make sure you get started with a skilled trainer to ensure that your technique is solid to minimize your risk of injury.

If you think that you eat in response to your daily stressors, start a primarily aerobic exercise routine; not as a means for weight loss, but rather as a stress relief tool. Whatever your needs are, selecting the proper type of exercise will maximize your chances of staying with it. Just like the other stations, the exercise regimen that you choose should become a permanent change to your daily routine.

Summary

- Moderate exercise is not enough to cause weight loss.
- Your goal for any exercise program should be to lower your set point by building muscle.
- For exercise, it's the intensity that matters, more so than the duration.
- Weight lifting and high intensity interval training make better choices than moderate cardiovascular exercise.
- Exercise should be your first option to help relieve stress.

Station 11 – Minimize Refined Oil

Limit your use of oil to 1-2 tablespoons daily. Limit your intake of any foods that contain oil (on the list of ingredients) to once per week. When cooking with oil, use only organic butter, palm, or coconut oil. Consider taking a fish oil supplement daily.

The popularity of the Mediterranean diet has tricked many of us into believing that olive oil is a healthy addition to our diet. Other oils, such as coconut and palm oil, have also been touted as "healthy" oils and their sales have sky rocketed as Americans search for a way to continue to eat rich, greasy foods with a clean conscience. Unfortunately, there is no such thing as "healthy" oil, just varying levels of unhealthy oils.

The Benefits of a Low Fat Diet

The benefits to your health of an extremely low fat diet are significant and have been touted by several influential physician-nutritionists such as Dean Ornish, MD and John McDougall, MD. They advocate a strict, vegan no-fat diet as the best method for weight loss and cardiovascular disease prevention. While their eating program does result in excellent weight loss, and is very effective for preventing and even reversing heart disease, many people have difficulty practicing this extremely strict eating style. Nonetheless, the health benefits of avoiding refined oils are significant and, if possible, should be practiced.

The profound impact of these extreme low-fat diets on cardiovascular disease can be amazing. There are hundreds of case reports of patients who were on the verge of needing cardiac surgery or even a heart transplant who were able to reverse their heart disease through diet alone. Former president, Bill Clinton, is a firm believer in the power of a low-fat vegan diet and started on this diet after undergoing multiple heart surgeries and angioplasties. The remarkable ability of an extremely low-fat diet to actually reverse heart disease proves the concept that there is no such thing as "heart healthy" oil; only some oils that cause less of a negative impact on your cardiovascular health than others.

However, there is still hope for those of us who find it too difficult to eliminate all refined oils completely. By eating a vegetable rich diet and limiting oil intake to 1-2 tablespoons daily, most of us can still achieve significant weight loss and cardiovascular disease prevention. Those individuals who have significant heart disease should aim to eliminate oils from their diet, or at the most, limit it to ½ tablespoon daily.

Although we will go into a detailed analysis of the healthfulness of many different oils, it's critical that you realize that none of the oils have any useful nutrients and all should be considered empty calories and avoided as much as possible. The differentiation between oils is based on the relative amount of harm that oils can cause your heart, arteries, and weight loss efforts, and not on their ability to positively impact your health. To some degree, all oils will raise your thermostat's set point; however, some will more than others. Oils are the most calorie dense of all foods, containing lots of calories and little to no nutrition. They are at the very end of our nutrient density spectrum and should be eaten sparingly.

Oils – The Temperature Matters

When considering the healthfulness of oils, one critical piece of information is necessary – whether or not the oil will be heated. Heating some oils causes significant degradation of the otherwise non-toxic mono and polyunsaturated components, especially if they are heated past their smoke point. In fact, many "healthy" oils break down and form dangerous trans-fats when they are heated while other "unhealthy" oils are much more heat stable. All of the data that supports the health benefits of olive oil is based on the intake of unheated, cold-pressed olive oil. It's very likely that there are absolutely no health benefits to a diet rich in olive oil if the oil is not cold pressed (meaning that it was heated during the extraction process) or used for cooking. To add to the confusion, the "unhealthy" saturated fats are much more heat stable and do not convert into dangerous trans-fats when they are heated.

The end result is that you should select different oils based on whether or not they will be heated. If you are using some of the less heat stable oils, keep the temperature as low as possible and pay careful attention that the oil does not smoke if you are using it for sautéing.

Best Oils for Cooking

- Organic or Amish Butter
- Coconut Oil
- Palm Oil

Best oils for non-heated use

- Extra Virgin Olive Oil
- Canola Oil
- Grapeseed Oil
- Walnut Oil
- Safflower Oil
- Sesame Oil
- Peanut Oil

Toxic Oils to Avoid

- Hydrogenated Oils
- Lard
- Margarine
- Partially Hydrogenated Oils
- Soybean Oil
- Corn Oil

Many people are surprised to see butter on the list of the best choices for cooking. If the cows are well cared for, the butter produced will be mostly saturated fats and will be very stable when cooked - making butter an excellent choice for cooking. Coconut Oil is the ideal cooking oil because it is extremely heat stable and is made up of much smaller fat molecules known as short and medium chain fatty acids.

Animal fats contain mostly the larger, long-chained fatty acids. Short and medium chain fatty acids are metabolized differently than the long chain fats and impact your thermostat and heart in a less damaging way. Also, butter from grass fed cows contains a much higher concentration of short and medium chain fatty acids than cows raised on grain and given hormones and antibiotics.

Palm Oil is also very heat stable but contains more of the mono and polyunsaturated fats that can break down during cooking; making it an acceptable, but not ideal, cooking oil choice. There is a lot of criticism pointed at the environmental impact of the palm oil industry since large sections of rain forest are being destroyed to make room for palm oil plantations. Given the availability of Amish butter and coconut oil, it's not necessary to use palm oil.

Olive Oil

Olive Oil has been widely touted as the healthiest oil and is used as a staple in most kitchens. While cold pressed, extra virgin olive oil served unheated does offer some health benefits compared to other oils, it still adds only a minimal amount of nutrition compared to the number of calories that it contains. Despite the polyphenols in olive oil that are thought to improve your cardiovascular health and the widespread popularity of the Mediterranean diet, olive oil is still a very calorie dense food and should be avoided. When olive oil is heated, the health benefits of the polyphenols are mostly destroyed and some of the oil is converted into a more dangerous form that will raise your thermostat's set point. Nonetheless, olive oil is more heat stable than many other oils and is an acceptable choice if not heated past the smoke point. Look for light olive oil which has a higher smoke point and makes a better choice for sautéing. When cooking with olive oil, try to minimize the heat and duration of cooking as much as possible.

When selecting oils for use in non-heated recipes, make sure you select cold pressed preparations. These preparations are not heated during the extraction process and therefore maintain the less damaging unsaturated components.

Many of the oils that are commonly used in processed food are unacceptable choices and will poison your thermostat. Hydrogenated and partially hydrogenated oils (trans-fats) raise your bad LDL cholesterol levels and lower your good HDL levels. Both of these changes result in a higher incidence of coronary artery disease. There is also a belief that trans-fats cause an increased risk of Alzheimer's disease, breast and prostate cancers, diabetes, fatty liver disease, and even depression. It's also clear that ounce for ounce, trans-fats will lead to more weight gain than other fats due to their thermostat raising effects.

Lard, margarine, corn, and soybean oils all contain very high amounts of omega-6 fatty acids. Most omega-6 fatty acids promote inflammation and therefore contribute to the development of arthritis, diabetes, cancer, and heart disease. Omega-6 oils also serve to raise your metabolic thermostat's set point.

At this point in the program, there are likely three different ways that you continue to consume refined oils:

1. As a salad dressing.
2. In processed foods.
3. As a cooking ingredient: typically while roasting vegetables or preparing animal proteins.

Let's look at each individually and identify ways to further minimize oil consumption.

Salad Dressing

Oil and vinegar is believed, by most, to be a very healthy

salad dressing because the oil is almost always olive oil which is a "healthy oil." Although selecting an oil and vinegar salad dressing is better than most of the commercially available salad dressings, the olive oil still contributes an unnecessary amount of calories to the salad. There are several better options than olive oil and vinegar salad dressing. Hopefully, you will be able to eliminate oil completely as a topping for your salad. You'll find that following the *Pound of Cure* eating plan strongly encourages you to eat a salad at least once a day. Your ability to find healthy, inexpensive, delicious salads that can be eaten without commercial salad dressing is critical for success. These concepts have been reviewed previously, but are worth repeating.

1) Eat the salad raw, using raw nuts and seeds as the flavor enhancer.
2) Use just vinegar (balsamic vinegar, red wine vinegar or a flavored vinegar).
3) Create your own salad dressing using one of our oil free recipes. These dressings use blended raw nuts and seeds as the primary component of the dressing instead of refined oils.

Processed Foods

Unfortunately, refined oils are present in most processed foods; even healthy, reduced calorie and organic selections. Processed foods require a long shelf life and refined oils are a very effective and inexpensive way to achieve this. Nonetheless, you have already limited your intake of processed foods significantly, so it's unlikely that you're receiving a large amount of oils from them.

Roasting vegetables

This is the most difficult place to eliminate oils from your diet and is the best place to use your 1-2 tablespoons per day. Nonetheless, there is still room for improvement in minimizing the amount of oils used for cooking. When cooking vegetables, first ask whether it is necessary that the vegetable be roasted. Steaming vegetables is an excellent method of preparation and can be done very easily with the help of a dedicated steamer. Vegetable steamers are inexpensive, easy to use and clean. You may find that steamed vegetables with added herbs and spices can be as delicious as vegetables roasted with oil. Add a few spritzes of olive oil to a plate of steamed vegetables after they're cooked. This allows you to further decrease the amount of oil that you use and ensures that the oil is not heated. Also water sautéing or "sweating" vegetables can be used in lieu of sautéing them in butter. If you must use oil, place it in a BPA-free spray bottle so that the oil can be dispersed evenly over the vegetables. Finally, animal proteins frequently require very little oil when cooking, and can often be delicious without any added oil at all. Experiment with poached and baked preparations of eggs and fish.

Although refined oils should be avoided as much as possible and even those marketed as "heart healthy" choices should be limited, there is one type of oil that we should actively try to add to our diet.

Omega 3 Fatty Acids

Ninety-nine percent of Americans are deficient in omega-3 fatty acids. These fats will lower your cholesterol and triglycerides, prevent heart disease, decrease inflammation in your blood vessels, and decrease your insulin levels. There is excellent evidence to support the fact that eating omega-3 fats will decrease your risk of developing breast, prostate, and colon cancer. The best way to increase your intake of omega-3 fats is in the form of supplements. However, eating small oily fish, grass fed beef, free-range organic eggs, and flaxseeds or flaxseed oil can allow you to become one of the one percent of Americans who take in enough of this vital nutrient. Since the price of wild caught fish can be 2-3 times more expensive than its farm-raised counterpart and may contain dangerously high levels of mercury, a much more affordable source of omega-3 fatty acids is smaller oily fish like anchovies, sardines, and herring. These are relatively inexpensive and do not have farm raised alternatives.

Flaxseed oil, also known as linseed oil, is a good source of omega-3 fatty acids. However, it is probably not as good of a choice as fish and animal based omega-3 sources. Flaxseed oil is edible but its strong flavor and odor may make you think otherwise. It smells and tastes as if it is better suited for its more common use – as a wood furniture finishing agent. Although flaxseed oil contains high amounts of omega-3 fatty acids, it comes in the form of Alpha-linolenic acid (ALA), rather than the more effective forms (EPA and DHA) which are found in fish oils. Our body is poorly suited for conversion of ALA to either EPA or DHA and it is likely that the same benefits that are provided by fish oil based omega-3 fatty acids are not conveyed by taking flaxseed oil supplements.

Fish Oil Supplements

The health benefits of omega-3 fatty acids are tremendous. It is difficult to get enough of these vital compounds in our diet due to the amount of pollution present in our oceans which limit our ability to safely eat wild fish. Because of this unfortunate fact, many people choose to take daily fish oil supplements. While this is an excellent choice, you should consider a few facts when choosing your supplement. First, avoid cod liver and shark oil supplements since toxins are concentrated in the liver of fish, making cod liver oils more likely to contain elevated levels of pollutants than other supplements. Sharks are predatory and therefore are subject to the principle of biomagnification in which the pollutants are concentrated at each level of the food chain, making the largest, predatory fish contain the highest concentration of pollutants.

Here are some guidelines in choosing a fish oil supplement.

1) It should contain omega-3 fatty acids, not just "fish oil."
2) It should list the amount of EPA and DHA (two omega-3 fatty acids) and the total amount of both should equal the total amount of oil in the product. If they don't add up, then this is a sign that it is a low quality supplement.
3) The fish oil should not be distilled – this can decrease the quality of the supplement significantly.

In this station, we will further minimize refined oils from our diet and further decrease the amount. Oils are the most calorie-dense foods on the planet and should be avoided as much as possible, even choices like olive oil and coconut oil. Depending on your weight loss and health goals, you should limit your intake of refined oils to between ½ and 2 tablespoons daily. Finally, consider carefully the oils used for cooking since heating oil changes the healthfulness significantly.

Summary

- All oils are unhealthy; the only difference between oils is how unhealthy they are.
- Heating oil past its smoke point can increase the harmfulness of the oil.
- When cooking with oils, choose a heat stable one.
- Consider taking a quality omega-3 fatty acid supplement.

Station 12 – Minimize Salt Intake

Minimize the amount of salt you add to non-vegetable food, either during or after preparation. It is acceptable to add a small amount of salt to vegetables. Limit cured meats and sausages to two servings per week.

Salt is a mineral – it is not a plant or animal as almost all the other food we eat is. There is absolutely no need to ingest salt directly in order to remain healthy – this is a common myth and absolutely untrue. You can lead a long healthy life and obtain enough sodium and chloride from the natural contents of food without ever adding a single grain of salt.

Since salt does not have calories, why is it important to keep salt intake to a minimum for weight loss purposes? Although salt will cause water weight gain, it does not promote or encourage the storage of fat. You will not store more fat simply by eating too much salt. It also does not have a significant effect on your metabolic thermostat. There are two reasons why eating salt will prevent you from meeting your weight loss goals. First, foods with high sodium content tend to be heavily processed, rich in refined carbohydrates, and high in calories. Second, salt is an appetite stimulant and will cause you to overeat salt seasoned foods (sometimes this can be used to your advantage). Salt should be kept to a minimum by anyone who has ever been diagnosed with high blood pressure.

How Much is Too Much?

A good rule of thumb for your daily intake of sodium is approximately 1 mg of Sodium for each calorie consumed. Most patients on the *Pound of Cure* eat between 1500 – 2000 calories daily (but who's counting?). Based on this caloric intake, you should limit your consumption of Sodium to 1500 – 2000 mg daily. The average American consumes over 3000 mg of Sodium every day, so you will be eating half the sodium of your friends and neighbors.

Even the healthy fruits and vegetables you eat contain sodium. However, it is almost impossible to take in too much sodium just from fruits and vegetables since they contain relatively small amounts. It is likely that your *Pound of Cure* eating plan will contain around 1000 mg of Sodium which leaves you 500 - 1000 mg (¼ - ½ of a teaspoon of table salt) to add directly to your vegetables, or to eat in condiments and cooking ingredients.

More than 75% of the salt consumed by the average American is already in the food that you eat, before you even lift the salt shaker. Salt is used by food manufacturers to prevent spoilage, disguise the metallic tastes of other additives and preservatives and to mask the dryness of foods like crackers, chips, and pretzels. Many familiar processed foods become practically inedible when they are prepared without salt. For instance, Corn Flakes® taste metallic when prepared without salt and Eggo waffles have been described as tasting like stale straw when the salt was left out.

Low-calorie, prepared meals are frequently the worst culprits, though breads, pizza, cold cuts, bacon, cheese, soups, and fast foods are also very high in sodium. Since these foods now play a very limited role in your diet, it's likely that you are already eating very little sodium. Based on these examples, it's clear that high sodium content is a marker for high fat and refined carbohydrate levels as well.

Cured Meats and Sausages

One group of foods that may still be present in your diet that likely contains too much sodium is cured meats like bacon and sausages. The wide availability of turkey bacon and lean sausages has made these foods commonplace in the diet of many *Pound of Cure* eaters for good reason since they are delicious, low in fat, easy to prepare, and add flavor to vegetable dishes. However, these foods have a lot of sodium. Turkey bacon contains 250 mg per slice and one small link of chicken sausage contains 200 mg. Although these foods are very useful adjuncts to your eating plan and can even be found in some of our recipes, they should be eaten no more than twice per week.

Eating cured meats and sausages can expose you to a dangerous group of chemicals called nitrosamines. Nitrosamines form when these foods react with the acid in your stomach. They are known carcinogens, though the amount necessary to cause healthy cells to become cancerous is unclear. Many scientists argue that the amount of exposure we get from eating these foods is not enough to cause cancer. Limiting these foods to two servings per week should keep you safe.

Salt and Your Appetite

Salt's role as an appetite stimulant is just being discovered. We've always known that eating high-salt foods will trigger thirst, but it's never been thought of as an appetite stimulant. Our brain's ability to separate thirst from hunger is not as good as we once thought. Frequently, we misinterpret thirst as hunger and overeat as a result. The clearest example of this phenomenon can be seen in people's nut consumption. Although raw, unsalted nuts are packed with nutrition and are very satiating, it is possible to overeat them which can impede your weight loss efforts. When eating raw nuts, a small handful is usually all that's necessary to satisfy your hunger. Eating salted nuts, typically does not provide the same degree of satiety.

Bitter and sweet tastes are hard wired into our DNA. Bitter tastes can denote a potentially poisonous food and our taste buds are predisposed to reject bitter foods. Sweet tastes historically represent a safe, nutritious food explaining why most of us prefer these foods over all others. Our predilection for salty tastes is not a preference that we are born with, but rather one we acquire - usually as a child. After maintaining the Pound of Cure diet for a significant amount of time, it is likely that your preference for salty tastes will diminish.

The one place where it's acceptable to add a little salt is on your roasted vegetables. Roasted vegetables are delicious, easy to make, and a great way to push your intake up to that magical two pound mark. Adding a little salt is likely to improve the taste and, of course, stimulate your appetite for more. It's worth the small amount of extra sodium to increase your enjoyment and desire for more vegetables. A small amount of salt added to roasted vegetables can be a strategic way to increase your consumption and should not be considered a violation of this station. Nonetheless, if you have no problem enjoying your vegetables without salt, there is no need to add some.

Finally, a high salt diet is a clear cause of high blood pressure and anyone who has ever been diagnosed with hypertension should ensure that they keep their daily sodium intake to 1500mg or less. African Americans appear to be particularly sensitive to the blood pressure raising effects of salt and should be extra vigilant. Because of the dangerous effects of high blood pressure on your heart, some estimate that if everyone in the United States followed a low sodium diet, we could save 150,000 lives every year.

Although sugar and fat contents have rightfully become the primary concern in processed foods, salt still plays an important role. Even though the *Pound of Cure* lifestyle is naturally low in salt, decreasing your salt intake can serve as the final finish to your new lifestyle.

Summary

- Try to keep your daily sodium intake to 1 mg per calorie consumed.
- Limit cured meats and sausages since they contain high levels of sodium.
- Salt can stimulate your appetite.

Conclusion

Following all 12 Stations of the *Pound of Cure* eating plan means that you will be eating a very different diet from the rest of your peers. It also means that your health will be very different and you won't be forced to endure the pain and suffering that diabetes, heart disease, high blood pressure, and arthritis brings. After years of working with patients on this program, I've learned that following all 12 Stations requires discipline and a strong commitment to change. When you are faced with severe medical illness and begin to see the results possible from this eating style, the discipline and motivation happens naturally. However, if you recognize that eliminating staples like bread and dairy from your diet is more than you're ready to take on, you can still make significant advances to your health by only following the first few stations.

Diet transformation is not something that should occur over night. I trust the longevity of a series of several small changes made over a year or even longer. I try to discourage my patients from making a complete and sudden change in their eating since this encourages an all or nothing mentality where you are either on the program or completely off - treading water until the next fad diet comes along.

If you feel overwhelmed at any point in the program, just stay where you are and don't put pressure on yourself to keep moving through to the last station. Overcommitting to change is one of the most common causes of weight loss failure and weight regain after a successful diet. If you need to move backward a station or two - this is acceptable - as long as you maintain some of the positive changes that you've made.

Before you get started, I recommend that you think about the reasons why you want to lose the weight and become healthier. As a physician, when I work with patients, it's always their high blood pressure, looming diabetes, or heart disease that motivates me to help them lose weight, knowing the pain and suffering that these diseases can result in. Often times, the patient has a completely different source of motivation. On a number of occasions, I've found a big smile on the face of a successful patient who has seemed unimpressed by their lower weight and improved health at past visits. When I inquire further, I often find stories of realized goals that have nothing to do with their health: such as riding a roller coaster for the first time in 15 years, going to a daddy-daughter dance, or riding on an airplane and not feeling self-conscious. I'm told that when they started their new lifestyle, they didn't want to tell me about these goals because it seemed trivial. Nothing could be further from the truth! Your reasons for losing weight should be embraced regardless of how others may perceive them. Identifying these sources of motivation and leaning on them when you are faced with temptations is a critical ingredient for long-term success.

Many patients start a weight loss program by setting goals such as "lose 20 pounds before the summer." I strongly discourage you from using the scale as a measure of your success or failure on this, or any other weight loss program. You are only in charge of the food choices that you make and the physical activities that you perform every day - not how your body responds to them. You may eat perfectly for weeks on end and for reasons we don't fully understand, the scale won't budge. Other times, you may have frequent indulgences and yet the scale shows you a few pounds lighter at the end of the week. Your daily weight is an unreliable measure of your adherence to the dietary and physical guidelines of this program. For this reason, I recommend you weigh yourself no more frequently than once per month, ideally only once per season. Weighing yourself more frequently only opens you up to the possibility of becoming frustrated with your short-term results and abandoning a program that would have ultimately resulted in long-term weight loss success.

Rather than specific weight loss goals, I recommend that you set goals that are completely within your control. For instance, if you want to push your weight loss further, set a goal that you exceed two pounds of vegetables every day for one week straight. Start the week off by making a big pot of vegetable soup and cutting up pounds of carrots, celery, cucumbers and peppers to snack on. In the end, whether you meet this goal will be completely under your control and is not subject to an external force like your body's finicky metabolism. When you start an exercise program, I recommend that you set goals based on your physical activities. Set a goal to jog a mile without stopping, compete in a 5K race, or even do 10 uninterrupted pushups.

Many people look at the restrictions of all 12 Stations and have trouble finding the motivation necessary to complete such a drastic lifestyle transformation. Thankfully, you do not need to make all of the changes at once. Just tackle each station as an individual goal with no time expectations of moving forward. Let the changes sink in and become part of your routine. You should not push yourself to move on to the next station until you are motivated to move forward. If you maintain your changes over several months comfortably but don't feel the need to push further, this should still be considered a success. Integrating even one of the stations into your life is a positive step and will improve your health. Most people never integrate all of the stations into their lives but still reap significant health benefits. If you are not ready for a drastic change, then don't make one. Make only small, manageable changes - slowly over time.

As you gradually improve your diet, it's important that you focus your improvements on the habits that count the most. Many people are hesitant to pursue a program like the *Pound of Cure* for fear that they won't be able to "enjoy life" and participate in the events that bring happiness: like evenings out at a restaurant or a family dinner. First, after you start eating well, you'll find that you are able to enjoy life more than ever. Second, the singular events that occur relatively infrequently like a special night out with your spouse or a holiday dinner have very little impact on your weight loss. These events occur at most once or twice a month and have a relatively insignificant impact on your diet and health. Rather than worrying about these special occasions and their impact on your health, you should focus your efforts on the things that you do every day. No one gained all their weight from eating too much of their own birthday cake – they only eat it once a year.

As you progress through the 12 Stations, my hope is that you will become more comfortable looking at the changes in your weight over the years as the result of alterations in your metabolic thermostat, rather than a failure or success of your willpower. Blaming yourself for your weight gain is a completely pointless exercise. Your weight gain was not caused by a lack of willpower and cannot be corrected by increasing it. There are many elaborate treatment programs designed to address your lack of control over eating. All of them will fail for the many reasons outlined in this book. In truth, a psychological disturbance is a very rare cause of weight gain. I often tell my patients that being crazy doesn't make you gain weight, but gaining weight can certainly make you crazy.

Decades ago, our medical community decided that obesity was the simple result of an excess of calories caused by the habits of gluttony and sloth. This viewpoint was soon widely adopted by the media and ultimately the rest of us. As I hope you've come to realize, there is no advice on weight loss that is less useful and more counter-productive than "eat less and exercise more." Let me be the first to apologize on behalf of doctors across the country for this misguided advice.

Our new thermostat based perspective on weight loss demonstrates that what you eat is much more important than how much you eat. I urge you to look at fruits and vegetables as the antidote to the poison that the American food chain delivers into your home. There has been a lot of criticism of the American food chain and its role in our country's obesity epidemic. Much of this criticism is rightfully directed. I urge those of you who feel passionate about misleading marketing claims and inhumane animal treatment in the food industry to join the many groups that are forming to address these problems.

Although these groups are important, it is unlikely that government intervention will provide the influence necessary to improve our nation's food supply. In the end, it will be the votes that are cast at the grocery store checkout counter and the tables at restaurants that will influence meaningful change. Cast your vote by boycotting commercial diet programs that emphasize portion control and starvation. Support restaurants and grocery stores that take great care in delivering whole, unprocessed foods to you. As Americans across the country decide that they would rather spend their money on healthy food than on prescription drugs and health insurance premiums, the food chain will adapt to meet this growing market. Vote with your fork, three times a day, and the world will listen.

In Health,

Matthew Weiner, MD, FACS

Recipes

Curried Cauliflower

- 1 head of cauliflower chopped to large bite sized pieces
- Pepper
- Curry powder
- Garlic powder
- 1 tablespoon of light olive oil in a spray bottle

Preheat oven to 425 degrees.

In a large mixing bowl (preferably with a top) season the cauliflower with a bit of pepper and garlic and then generously apply the curry so the cauliflower is well coated. Cover the bowl and shake it. Spread your cauliflower on a lightly spritzed baking sheet and roast uncovered for 20 minutes until the cauliflower is tender. You can add a few extra spritzes of olive oil to the dish before serving.

Butternut Squash, Basil and Pumpkin Seeds

- 1 lb. butternut squash peeled and chopped into large bite size pieces
- 1 tablespoon of light olive oil in a spray bottle
- Salt
- Pepper
- Garlic
- 2 ounces of pumpkin seeds

In a large mixing bowl spritz olive oil over the butternut squash and mix thoroughly until fully coated. Add the pumpkin seeds in. Season with salt, pepper, and garlic to taste and roast in a 425-degree oven for 20- 25 minutes until tender and caramelized.

Burrito Salad

- Shredded romaine lettuce
- Chopped black olives
- Avocado and/or guacamole
- Chopped tomatoes
- Chopped onions
- Chopped peppers
- Fresh Salsa
- 3-4 oz. per person of turkey meat, chicken breast, or steak
- Chili powder
- Cilantro
- Spray bottle of light olive oil
- Black or pinto beans
- Chick peas

Sauté onions in a nonstick frying pan sprayed lightly with olive oil to prevent sticking and allow them to caramelize.

After 5 minutes, add the peppers and cook for an additional 5 minutes. Next add whatever protein source you choose and sauté until cooked through (if using steak sauté to your desired taste). Place in serving bowl. Generously add remaining ingredients to mixture and serve over the shredded romaine.

Brussels Sprouts with Mustard and Turkey Bacon

- 1 ½ pounds of Brussels sprouts cut in half
- 5 Spritzes of light olive oil
- 5 Slices turkey bacon
- 2 Teaspoons Dijon mustard
- 2 Tablespoons capers
- 1 Tablespoon lemon juice
- 6 anchovies minced
- Pepper and garlic to taste

Roast Brussels sprouts without oil at 425 degrees for 15 minutes. While Brussels sprouts are roasting, sauté your turkey bacon in a non-stick pan at a low temperature. When bacon is crispy, crumble, and mix the Brussels sprouts with all of the other ingredients (including the olive oil spritzes). Return to oven for 5 minutes.

Sugar Snap Peas

- 1 lb. sugar snap peas
- 8 or 9 spritzes of sesame oil
- 1 tablespoon of black sesame seeds
- Salt and pepper to taste

Trim the stringy ends from the peas. Mix all ingredients together and serve cold or at room temperature. This makes a great snack between meals.

Guacamole

- 3 peeled and quartered avocados
- 1 teaspoon lime juice
- Salt pepper to taste
- Spritz bottle of light olive oil
- 1 cup butternut squash cut in small cubes
- Cilantro to taste

Spritz the olive oil over the butternut squash and bake at 415 degrees for 22 minutes. Cool in refrigerator for 20 minutes. Chop avocado and lightly mash. Season with salt, pepper, cilantro, and lime. Mix in butternut squash carefully to retain chunkiness. Perfect for lunch mixed with 1-2 cups of chopped cucumbers.

Carrot Ginger Soup

- 2 lbs. of carrots
- 1 bunch of celery
- 1 medium onion
- 4 tablespoons minced ginger
- 1 cup almond milk or coconut milk
- 2 cooked chicken breasts minced
- 1 tablespoon of Light olive oil
- 48 oz. chicken stock
- Season to taste with curry, salt, pepper, and garlic powder

Puree carrots, onion and celery in a food processor and combine it in a pot with chicken stock and almond/ coconut milk. Cook covered on medium heat until carrot bits are soft and cooked through. Add ginger and keep cooking for one hour. Season with salt, pepper, curry and garlic to taste. Remove from heat, add minced chicken breasts, and stir well.

Cauliflower Soup

- Light olive oil
- 1 medium onion sliced thin
- 1 whole cauliflower broken into florets
- 5 cups water
- Salt and black pepper to taste

Spritz a heavy-bottomed pan with olive oil and sweat the onions over low heat for 15 minute without letting it brown. Add the cauliflower and 1/2 cup water. Raise the heat slightly, cover the pot tightly, and simmer the cauliflower for 15 to 18 minutes, or until tender. Add another 4 1/2 cups hot water; bring to a low simmer and cook an additional 20 minutes uncovered.

Working in batches, purée the soup in a blender to a very smooth, creamy consistency. Let the soup stand for 20 minutes which will allow it to thicken slightly. Thin the soup with an additional ½ cup of hot water. Reheat the soup. Serve hot, seasoned with salt and freshly ground black pepper.

Salad Nicoise

- 1 bag of washed mixed salad greens
- 1/2 cup trimmed green beans
- 1/3 cup of Nicoise olives
- 1 cup chopped tomatoes
- 2 soft boiled eggs sliced thin
- 1 tablespoon of capers
- salt, pepper, and garlic powder to taste
- Light olive oil
- 8-Ounce piece of tuna or salmon.

Spray fish on each side with olive oil and season with salt, pepper and garlic powder. Sauté in a hot pan on each side for 5-7 minutes until the fish is the temperature you prefer. Remove the fish from heat and let sit for 5 minutes before slicing. Mix all other ingredients together. No dressing is required since the liquid from the tomatoes, olives and soft boiled yolk will create a salad dressing effect. Cut the fish in half and arrange on top of the salad and serve.

Cream of Broccoli Soup

- Light olive oil
- 1 medium onion sliced thin
- 1 head fresh cauliflower broken into florets
- 1 head of roasted broccoli chopped
- 5 cups of water
- Salt and freshly ground black pepper to taste

Spray the onion with the olive oil and sweat over low heat without letting it brown for approximately 15 minutes. Roast the broccoli by spraying it with the olive oil and baking at 400 degrees for twenty minutes. After the broccoli is roasted, puree it in a food processor (leave a few chunks). In a saucepan, add the cauliflower to the broccoli, salt to taste, and add 1/2 cup water. Raise the heat slightly, cover the pot tightly, and stew the cauliflower for 15 to 18 minutes, or until tender. Then add another 4 1/2 cups hot water, bring to a low simmer and cook an additional 20 minutes uncovered. Working in batches, purée the soup in a blender to a very smooth, creamy consistency. Let the soup stand for 20 minutes. In this time it will thicken slightly.
Thin the soup with 1/2 cup hot water. Reheat the soup. Serve hot, seasoned to taste with salt and freshly ground black pepper.

Brazilian Black Bean Soup

- Light olive oil
- 3 cups onion, chopped
- 10 cloves garlic, crushed
- 2 teaspoons cumin
- 2 teaspoons salt
- 1 medium carrot, diced
- 1 medium red bell pepper, diced
- 30 oz. black beans, drained
- 1 1/2 cups of orange juice
- 2 medium tomatoes, diced
- 2 cups of frozen corn
- 1 bunch of fresh cilantro (to taste)
- Black and cayenne pepper (to taste)

In a stockpot spray oil on onions, garlic, cumin, salt and carrots. Stir over medium heat until carrots are just tender. Add the peppers and sauté everything until tender (another 10-15 min). Add the rest of the ingredients. Puree half of the soup with a blender. Simmer for 15 min. Serve with fresh cilantro.

Chinese Chicken Salad

- 1 pound of organic free range chicken cutlets
- 2 broccoli crowns cut into bite sized pieces
- 1 pound of fresh Brussels sprouts shredded
- 1 pound of sugar snap peas trimmed
- 1 cup of frozen peas thawed
- 1 cup of shredded carrots
- 1 cup of bean sprouts
- Sesame oil in a spritz bottle
- Light olive oil
- 1 tablespoon of sesame seeds
- Pepper and garlic powder to taste
- Use Japanese Ginger, Asian Peanut or Shogun dressing (recipe listed below)

Preheat oven to 325 degrees. Combine Brussels sprouts, broccoli and shredded carrots in a large mixing bowl with a lid. Spread Brussels sprouts, broccoli and carrots on 2 large baking sheets and roast for 20 minutes. After cooking set aside to cool and add a few spritzes of sesame oil.

Lightly spritz your chicken breast with olive oil, season with pepper and garlic and sauté in a pan until thoroughly cooked and set aside.

When cooled, slice the chicken into thin strips and add to the mixture. Add the snap peas, bean sprouts and thawed green peas. Dress each serving, sprinkle with sesame seeds and serve at room temperature or chilled.

Vegetarian Chili

- 1 cup coarsely chopped onion
- ½ cup celery, rinsed and chopped
- 1 cup green bell pepper, rinsed and diced
- 1 can of black beans, drained and rinsed
- 1 can of red kidney beans, drained and rinsed
- 1 can of pinto beans, drained and rinsed
- 1 teaspoon ground cumin
- 1 teaspoon chili powder
- Light olive oil
- 1 can (16 oz.) of stewed tomatoes

In an 8-quart stockpot, spray the olive oil on the bottom of the pan and heat to medium. Add onion and cook and stir until onion starts to soften (usually about 5 minutes). Add celery and green pepper. Cook and stir another 5 minutes, until all vegetables soften. Add drained and rinsed beans to pot and stir in tomatoes, cumin, and chili powder. Bring to a boil, cover, reduce heat, and simmer 10–20 minutes to blend flavors.

Bean Soup

- 6 stalks celery diced
- 3 large carrots diced
- 2 large onions diced
- 1 pound dry navy beans (soak overnight)
- 2 large cans College Inn chicken broth
- 1 small can tomato paste
- Light olive oil
- Salt and pepper to taste

Put all the vegetables in large stockpot. Spray with olive oil and sauté until softened. Add rest of ingredients and simmer at low heat for 2-3 hours.

Gazpacho

- 2 large cans of tomato juice
- 2 large cucumbers with peel cut into 1" slices
- 2 large green peppers cut into large pieces
- 8 plum tomatoes quartered
- 2 red onions peeled and quartered
- 2-3 cloves of garlic, mashed
- Salt, black and cayenne pepper to taste
- ½ cup red wine vinegar

Use a food processor to chop each vegetable individually leaving some chunkiness. Combine the vegetables with tomato juice, red wine vinegar and seasoning and combine well. Chill. May be kept in refrigerator for several days.

Lentil Soup

- 5 carrots
- 1 medium-large onion
- 1 pound red lentils rinsed well-do not soak
- 64 ounces of chicken broth
- Light olive oil
- salt and pepper
- cumin
- bay leaf
- fresh lemon

Chop carrots and onions in a food processor, just short of puree. Spray with olive oil and sauté in a stockpot. Add in

the lentils and broth. Bring to a boil and add seasoning.
Simmer approximately 2 hours or until thickened and serve
with fresh lemon slices.

Hamburger Salad

- 1 package of mixed greens.
- 4 tomatoes chopped
- 1 yellow onion chopped
- 2 sliced Portobello mushrooms
- 1 ripe avocado sliced
- 4 ounces of organic lean grass fed ground beef per person
- Light olive oil
- Pickles
- Ketchup
- Mustard
- Pepper
- Garlic powder

Toss tomatoes, avocado and greens in a large mixing bowl.
Spray onions with olive oil and sauté over a medium flame,
stirring until they begin to brown and start to turn
translucent. Add the mushrooms to the pan, stirring to ensure
things are browning but not burning. Add ground meat to
the pan in pieces approximately 1 tablespoon in size. Season
the mixture with pepper and garlic. Remove from heat and
drain off any extra liquid with a strainer. Add the meat,
onions, and mushrooms to the salad and lightly toss. Serve
immediately with ketchup, mustard, and pickles.

Shrimp Salad

- 1 can hearts of palm cut into uniform coins
- 1 can of artichoke hearts chopped into bite sized pieces
- 2 ripe avocados cubed into bite sized pieces
- 3 or 4 medium tomatoes chopped into bite sized pieces
- 8 oz. of chilled steamed shrimp chopped into bite sized pieces
- Salt and pepper to taste

Mix all ingredients and serve chilled

Steak Salad

- 4 oz. of grass fed tenderloin per person
- Mixed greens
- Sliced tomatoes
- Chopped cucumbers
- Chick peas
- Sautéed red onions
- Salt, pepper and garlic powder to taste
- Horseradish Sauce (see recipe below)

Add the salt, pepper and garlic powder to the steak and cook it on the grill to desired temperature. Slice the steak and mix it with the rest of the ingredients. Top with the horseradish sauce and serve.

Egg "Salad"

- 1 very small pad of butter
- 1 handful of arugula
- 1 handful of frisee
- 2 eggs (farm fresh if possible)

Place the butter in a frying pan and melt it. Sautee the arugula completely. Place the Frisee in for 30 seconds. Place the arugula and frisee on the plate. Cook the eggs over easy. Serve the eggs on top of the frisee and Arugula.

Chocolate Peanut Butter Banana Ice Cream

- 4 frozen ripe bananas (freeze overnight)
- 2 ounces of 100 % Natural Peanut butter
- 2 tablespoons of unsweetened Cocoa powder

Blend until creamy. It doesn't taste as good as ice cream - it tastes better.

Nut Based Salad Dressings

Asian Peanut Salad Dressing

- 4 tablespoons of creamy 100% natural peanut butter
- 3 tablespoons of rice vinegar
- 3 tablespoons of water
- 1 tablespoon of low sodium soy sauce
- ½ clove of garlic
- 1 tablespoon of peeled ginger root
- 1 teaspoon of crushed red pepper flakes

Place all ingredients into a blender or food processor and puree. Serve over your favorite salad.

Presto Pesto Salad Dressing

- ½ cup of pine nuts
- ½ cup of fresh basil
- 2 tablespoons of balsamic vinegar
- 4 tablespoons of water
- Garlic to taste
- Salt
- Pepper

Place pine nuts, basil, vinegar, garlic and water into a blender or food processor and blend until smooth. Add salt and pepper to taste. Serve over your favorite salad instead of a Vinaigrette or Italian dressing.

Japanese Ginger Salad Dressing

- ¼ cup of canned coconut milk
- 3 tablespoons of rice vinegar
- ½ cup of raw cashews
- 1 tablespoon of miso paste
- 1 teaspoon of fresh, peeled chopped ginger

Place all the ingredients in a food processor and blend until smooth. Serve over your favorite salad

Shogun Dressing

- ½ cup almond milk
- ¼ cup chick peas
- 1 cup of baby carrots
- ¼ cup of pine nuts
- 1 tablespoon of rice vinegar
- 2 teaspoons of ginger root, peeled
- 1 tablespoon of shredded coconut (optional)

Place all the ingredients in a food processor and blend until smooth. Serve over your favorite salad

Creamy Caesar Dressing

- 1 tablespoon of Dijon mustard
- ½ cup of canned coconut milk
- ½ cup of garbanzo beans
- 1 teaspoon of capers
- 1 tablespoon of shelled pistachios
- 3 anchovies minced (optional)

Place all the ingredients in a food processor or blender and puree until smooth. Use in place of Caesar dressing or as a vegetable dip.

Athena Dressing

- 1 clove of garlic
- ½ teaspoon of salt (optional)
- 2 teaspoons of Dijon mustard
- 1 tablespoon of lemon juice
- 5 tablespoons of red wine vinegar
- 1 teaspoon of basil leaves
- ½ teaspoon of oregano leaves
- ½ cup of unsweetened almond milk
- ½ cup of chick peas
- ½ cup of pine nuts

Place all the ingredients in a food processor and blend until smooth. Serve over a Greek style salad.

Horseradish Sauce

- ½ cup of almond milk
- 2 tablespoons of sautéed onions
- ¼ cup of pine nuts
- ¼ cup of chick peas
- 2 tablespoons of horseradish root
- 1 tablespoon of distilled white vinegar
- Salt to taste

Place all the ingredients in a food processor and blend until smooth. Serve over a steak salad.

Set Point Smoothies

Before getting started with your set point smoothies, you will need a blender. Most of the more expensive models will pulverize the greens more effectively and will not burn out the motor the way the less expensive models may. If you are serious about smoothies (remember, they are the most potent of all set point lowering foods) then an investment in a quality blender will be worth the money.

Green Monster Smoothie

- 1 bunch of dandelion greens
- 1/3 of a pineapple cut up into 1" pieces
- 2" piece of ginger root (to taste)
- Ice

Blend until smooth.

Greena Colada

- 1 small bunch of kale
- 1 banana
- 2 tablespoons of dried coconut flakes (unsweetened)
- 1 cup of coconut milk
- Cilantro to taste
- Ice

Blend into a cool drink.

Green Apple Smoothie

- 1 apple
- 2 carrots
- 4 one inch slices of cucumber
- 1 cup of spinach
- 1 cup of ice
- 8 ounces of water

Blend until smooth.

Beginner's Smoothie

- ½ cup of frozen strawberries
- ½ cup of frozen mango
- 1 banana
- 1 cup of ice
- ½ cup of water
- 2 cups of baby spinach

Blend until smooth

Wake Me Up Smoothie

- 1 banana
- 1 large orange
- 2 bags of green tea
- 1 teaspoon of fresh ginger
- 2 cups of baby spinach

Open the tea bags and empty the contents into a blender with the rest of the ingredients. Blend until smooth. This smoothie will contain as much caffeine as a cup of coffee, so avoid drinking it in the evening if you have trouble sleeping.

Parsley Grapefruit Smoothie

- 1 grapefruit, peeled
- 2 cups of fresh parsley
- 1 cup of ice

Blend until smooth

30887605R00085

Made in the USA
Middletown, DE
10 April 2016

"I lost 45 pounds and never felt hungry! I finally know how to make healthy food choices, I have more energy and I'm more active than I've been in years. Thank you Dr. Weiner!"

"I've finally figured out why I've struggled with my weight my whole life and now have a clear plan."

"I felt like I was eating all the time, but the weight kept coming off."

"This book is the conversation about my weight that I've always wanted to have with my doctor."

A Pound of Cure was written by *Dr. Matthew Weiner*, a bariatric surgeon who has identified a style of eating that can bring about the same metabolic changes seen after gastric bypass surgery. The shifts in your metabolism that block hunger and prevent weight loss plateaus after surgery can be obtained by focusing your diet on nutrient rich foods like fruits and vegetables. The style of eating outlined shows you how to use food to control hunger, eliminate cravings and prevent a slow down in your metabolism that plagues typical starvation diets.

A Pound of Cure is a step by step guide that shows you how to change your style of eating sensibly, over time. Each of the 12 changes, or "stations" outlined in the program brings you closer to gaining control over the hunger and food cravings that have sabotaged your previous efforts. It is designed to be a lifelong change and nothing less and does not buy into the madness of starvation or fad diets.

If you are tired of the fad diets and the commercial diet industry that peddles artificial, synthetic diet foods as healthy choices, the *Pound of Cure* plan will show you how to eat sensibly, control your hunger and lose the weight for the rest of your life.

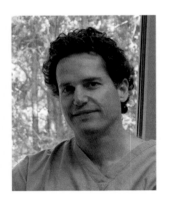

Matthew Weiner, MD is a weight loss surgeon who lives and practices in the suburbs of Detroit, Michigan. He performs gastric bypass, gastric sleeve and gastric banding surgery as well as offering non-surgical weight loss assistance in his practice. Dr. Weiner completed his medical degree from the University of Michigan and did his residency training at New York University. He is passionate about nutrition and its critical role in our health and well-being. He is an avid tennis player and happily married father of two little girls.

"What station are you on?"

ISBN 9781481061148

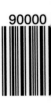